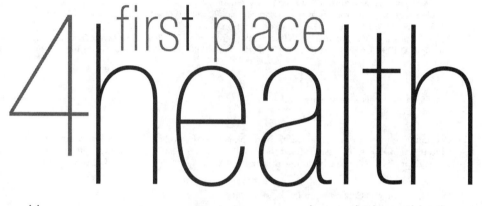

first place 4 health

discover a new way to healthy living

CAROLE LEWIS

with MARCUS BROTHERTON

Published by Regal
From Gospel Light
Ventura, California, U.S.A.
www.regalbooks.com
Printed in the U.S.A.

Caution: The information contained in this book is intended to be solely for informational and educational purposes. It is assumed that the First Place 4 Health participant will consult a medical or health professional before beginning this or any other weight-loss or physical fitness program.

Library of Congress Cataloging-in-Publication Data
Lewis, Carole, 1942-
First place 4 health / Carole Lewis with Marcus Brotherton.
    p. cm.
ISBN 978-0-8307-4523-4 (hard cover)
1. Spiritual life—Christianity. 2. Weight loss—Religious aspects—Christianity. I. Brotherton, Marcus. II. Title.
BV4501.3.L495 2008
613.2'5—dc22
                                                                            2007039835

1 2 3 4 5 6 7 8 9 10 / 10 09 08

Rights for publishing this book outside the U.S.A. or in non-English languages are administered by Gospel Light Worldwide, an international not-for-profit ministry. For additional information, please visit www.glww.org, email info@glww.org, or write to Gospel Light Worldwide, 1957 Eastman Avenue, Ventura, CA 93003, U.S.A.

contents

Part 1: Heart
Seeking Balance Emotionally

Part 2: Soul
Seeking Balance Spiritually

Part 3: Mind
Seeking Balance Mentally

Part 4: Strength
Seeking Balance Physically

Acknowledgments

I want to thank the many people who have worked so hard to bring the First Place 4 Health program to the place it is today. When the original First Place program began in March 1981, there were many people who were instrumental in seeing that the fledgling program got off to a great start. Special thanks to:

- Dottie Brewer, founder of the program

- Marilyn Stelley, who faithfully typed all the first manuscripts

- Buddy Griffin, minister of activities in 1981, who believed so strongly in the program that he went to bat to make it become a reality

- Kelly Roberts, who wrote the very first Bible study

- Barbara Grogan, Lois McCall, Dr. William Heston, Sally Johnson, Susan Crawford, Bobby Boyles, Beth Moore, Denise Munton, June Chapko, Martha Rogers, Susan Sowell and Elizabeth Crews, each of whom authored the Bible studies that followed

- Our First Place 4 Health staff in Houston, both past and present, whose prayers and support are evidence of the wonderful blessings that happen in the workplace when Christ is given first place

Finally, I want to take this opportunity to say thank you to everyone who has contributed to the growth of the First Place 4 Health program. It would take pages and pages to list every person who has worked untold hours for God's glory. If you are one of the thousands of First Place 4 Health members or leaders, please accept our heartfelt gratitude for all you have done to make this the finest total health program in existence today.

A History of Caring

Early in 1980, 12 men and women began to pray.

Knowing that God is interested in everything that concerns His children, they prayed that God would help them create a program to help them lose weight and find balance in every area of life—spiritually, mentally, emotionally and physically. These men and women were members of Houston's First Baptist Church, a congregation of about 20,000 members, located in Houston, Texas. They also knew in their hearts the importance of waiting on God for His perfect program in His perfect time.

They decided on a name for the program based on Matthew 6:33: "But seek first His kingdom and His righteousness, and all these things will be given to you as well." From that verse came the name *First Place*, with the understanding that any success we have, in any area of life, comes by putting Christ first.

The idea of creating a program around a balanced life came from the words of Jesus in Mark 12:30: "Love the Lord your God with all your heart, with all your soul, with all your mind and with all your strength."

In the beginning, everything started out small. One person wrote the First Place Bible study; another designed the notebook with a bright yellow cover and blue print. Dotty Brewer created all the forms to be used in the program because she was the most organized member of the group. First Place was officially launched in March 1981. I became a member of that first group.

People at First Baptist Church responded well to the program. Word got around, and by 1983, other churches were beginning to ask for the First Place program. Those who had completed First Place and moved to other churches were asking, "How can we do First Place at our new church? This is too wonderful to give up."

Dotty Brewer, the founder of the program, presented First Place to a publisher in Dallas and proposed selling the program to them. They wanted to make it available to the public through Christian bookstores. On her way back to Houston, however, as Dotty was praying, she felt God impressing her to keep the program at First Baptist Church and train people to use the materials. She felt convinced that people would not know what to do with the materials unless they were taught how to use them, and they would not realize how important group support is to success in the program.

The decision was made that First Place would remain in the church. The 12 men and women involved in the original writing of First Place had the program copyrighted, and they signed their copyright over to Houston's First Baptist Church. Their desire was for the First Place program to always be a ministry of the church. In 1986, we began to officially offer the program to other churches. People responded well, and Dotty and I began traveling to different states to teach leaders how to love and care about people through leading a First Place group.

By July 1987, First Place was being used in approximately 50 churches. At about that same time, Dotty Brewer approached me about taking over the program. Dotty was confident that I loved First Place and that my relationship with God had grown to the point where she felt that she could step back and turn the program over to me. Dotty left some big shoes to fill when I became the director of First Place. I will always admire her for the many ways she contributed to the launching of the program.

Those first few months in my new role were hectic. I took all the orders by phone and opened all the new accounts. I shipped a lot of the materials. I did the billing each month. I knew everyone who had an account with First Place and handled every facet of the work. It was a wonderful job! As the program grew, I was learning more and more about the heart and soul of First Place. But life was about to change again, in a big way.

Growing Through Change

God knew that when I began directing First Place in the summer of 1987, Dotty was going to become ill in the fall of that same year.

In July 1988, Dotty was diagnosed with colon cancer and lived for eight months after the diagnosis. I spent many hours at Dotty's bedside, along with Kay Smith, who later became my associate at First Place. Whenever Dotty wanted us with her at the hospital, we were there. Little did we know how God was preparing us for the tasks ahead.

At night, as I sat with Dotty and read her prayer journal, I learned that she was a person who consistently prayed for others. God allowed me to see the depth of her spirit.

God worked in my own heart during this time of pain and grief as I watched Dotty's body deteriorate. Her body was wasting away, but her heart was still strong because she had been an exercise walker for 15 years. It made me rethink my own exercise program, because Dotty had always joked about the fact that if she ever got sick God was going to have to beat her heart to death with a stick! Did I really want my heart to outlive my body? I realized that our days are in the Lord's hands, and none of us is going to leave this body ahead of the time He has planned. But until that time comes, we need to be good stewards of the body God has given us.

Dotty went home to be with the Lord on March 22, 1989. I'll never forget something she said about three weeks before she died. Though she was very sick, she never lost her sense of humor. Propped up on some pillows, and knowing that she wasn't going to live much longer, she said, "Carole, of all people, I would never have chosen you as director of First Place." We had a good laugh and talked about what a sense of humor God has.

The reason Dotty made this statement was that she had experienced firsthand what a rebel I was, in 1981, when we first met. I remember trying to fill out my Food Diary most weeks right before our First Place leader's meeting began. Dotty would say, "It's kind of hard to remember what you ate a week ago. Wouldn't it be easier to write it down when you eat it?"

It was only through God (and nothing that I did) that First Place soon grew from 50 groups to more than 1,200 groups in churches throughout the United States.

In 1990, we were approached by LifeWay Christian Resources of the Southern Baptist Convention about the possibility of their becoming the publisher for First Place. We had gone from printing the program in our own print shop and having our First Place leaders put the notebooks together, to hiring outside printers to do the job. This seemed like the next logical step. As we prayed together, it became evident that this was God's plan for the future of the program.

We revised the original program, adding a cookbook and a prayer journal, to introduce First Place through LifeWay in the summer of 1991. From 1991 until 1999, the program grew rapidly, with more than 12,000 groups meeting in the United States and in more than 15 foreign countries.

In 1999, we began looking for a publisher who would enable us to present the program to other denominations and a greater number of bookstores. We had felt secure and sheltered within our own denomination, so our prayer was that God would not let us make a mistake in choosing a new publisher. He answered our prayer, and in the summer of 2000, we were invited to visit Gospel Light in Ventura, California, to talk about a partnership.

Gospel Light had prayed for two years for a new adult curriculum program, and we at First Place had been praying for two years that God would guide us to the right publisher. In October 2000, Gospel Light became the publisher of First Place resources.

In July 2001, First Place was introduced at the annual CBA (Christian Booksellers Association convention)—now called ICRS (International Christian Retail Show). Since that time, the First Place materials have been available for purchase in bookstores and on the Internet, and several of our books have been published in different languages.

At the writing of these words, First Place is undergoing its third major revision, which includes a name change to First Place 4 Health. We are excited about what God has planned for the future of the program!

God often chooses unlikely people to serve Him, but He is more than able to take any one of us and do great and mighty things through us. From the time we accept Jesus as our personal Savior, God promises never to leave us. We may attempt to control our own lives for a period of time—maybe even for years—but we have the assurance that the Holy Spirit is continually working to mold us into the person God created us to be.

Beginning Your Journey

I'm so glad that you have chosen First Place 4 Health as the starting place to know that God will be with you in every choice you make, if you let Him. As you begin your journey, you may not realize all that is changing in your life until much later. But eventually you will know without a doubt that God has been with you from the very beginning.

He helped me choose a direction that has resulted in lasting positive changes in my life. I'm confident that He will do the same for you.

Carole Lewis
Houston, Texas

Just Give Us a Year

Many of us love for things to stay the same. We find comfort in the predictability of our routines. We let the dog out every night just before we go to bed. We look for our slippers in the same place every morning. We set the coffee pot to brew six cups of coffee by 6:30 A.M. What falls in between, well—it would be just fine if nothing ever got shaken, shattered or shimmied out of order.

But here's an unalterable truth about life: Change happens whether we like it or not.

We absolutely cannot stop things from changing. It's time to get a haircut again. Our preferred brand of cereal is no longer being sold. Our favorite pastor retires. People get jobs and lose jobs. Friends move into our lives for a season and then are gone. Kids grow up and become adults. After fall comes winter; after winter comes spring.

The truth is, even though many of us like things to stay the same, we secretly wish things were different—*very* different. When we scratch just below the surface of our comfortable routines, we wish the changes that happened to us were only positive changes—ones that foster our health, wholeness and healing. Things like . . .

- We wish we had more energy.
- We wish we looked good in our clothes.
- We wish we were a better parent, a better spouse, a better employee, a better leader, a better friend.
- We wish we could look in the mirror and like who we see.

As much as we might say that we like things to stay the same, on the inside we actually long for change. Real change. Beneficial change. Lasting change.

In our core, we long to be the people God has called us to be. We long to live the abundant life Christ talks about in John 10:10.

The problem is that we don't know how to change for the better. Maybe we don't even know how to get started.

Oh sure, we've tried making positive changes in the past, especially when it comes to health. We know what we need to do. We need to lose weight; we need to exercise. We need to dress for success and stay tan and get waxed and be empowered and leap and jump and fly off of tall buildings with a single bound and do everything every book, speaker, magazine article and grocery store tabloid ever tells us we absolutely must do and be to succeed.

We've heard it all. In fact, we've been bombarded with so much information about what we need to do and be that when we think about making any changes the thought just makes us tired.

There are moments when we feel helpless to change. We feel hopeless, guilt-ridden and full of shame. And we seriously doubt that things will ever be different.

One of the most important truths I've learned during the past 21 years as director of First Place 4 Health is that change is a given. We will either change for the better or for the worse, but we will change. I also know that we have a choice when it comes to every positive change in our life, and until we make that choice, we are still changing—but not for the better.

These are the cold, hard facts. I won't lie to you. I won't tell you that beneficial change is overly easy or that all positive change is completely pain-free, or that dramatic, positive changes happen overnight, or that you can run marathons by next week, even though you can't climb a flight of stairs today.

But I will tell you this: You can do it! You can change for the better. You can get started today on the road to living the life you were meant to live.

You can begin today to find balance in all areas of your life. The fullness of a balanced life brings wholeness.

And balanced life is well within your reach.

The Largest Recliner Available

My good friend Bev Henson once weighed nearly 320 pounds.

She never thought she'd weigh that much. None of us ever plan to be overweight. But change had come to her life. Not negative change at first. Just change. How she responded began the long, slow downhill slide.

In college, Bev was a competitive swimmer. She had the body of an athlete; she was good at swimming and she was dedicated and capable. She trained and practiced and worked toward her goals.

She also ate like an athlete. But with the amount of working out she did, she never had to worry about her weight.

When she graduated from college, her swimming ended. In those days there was no place for a good amateur swimmer to go, so Bev simply stopped. But she kept eating the way she had always eaten.

By age 34, Bev's weight had taken over her body. She hated how she looked and felt. She tried every weight-loss program available, but none seemed to work for long. She made several attempts to get her life under control—some serious, some almost far-fetched.

Once, a faith healer came to town. Bev was convinced that this was the answer to her weight problem. She talked it up with a bunch of women from her church. She rented a bus, and they raced over to see the healer.

One problem: He was only healing people in wheelchairs that night.

About that time, Bev grew resigned to living in poor health. Change had brought her a life she never thought she would ever lead. What else was there to do now but go out and buy the largest recliner she could find? So that's what she did. And there she sat. And there she stayed.

One New Year's Eve, Bev was reading her Bible when she encountered Zechariah 4:6: "Not by might, nor by power, but by my Spirit, says the LORD Almighty." She came across the name Zerubbabel. This is the man who had taken a strong leadership role in the rebuilding of the Temple that had been destroyed by Babylon 70 years earlier (read his story in Ezra 2-4). Before Zerubbabel and the rest of the Temple builders laid the foundation of the Temple, he had surveyed the ruins of the Temple site and wondered how it could ever be rebuilt. Yet he did not give in to the opposition around him.

Bev prayed that God would accomplish a similar attitude change in her own life. She did not see how she would ever be able to return to the health of her earlier days, but she wanted to try. She wanted to do it for the Lord, and she wanted to do it right.

This prayer was just one step in the right direction . . . just one positive change. But it got the ball rolling.

"God changed everything about me," Bev says today.

Now, at age 54, Bev has lost 150 pounds. She kayaks, runs, bikes and works as a personal trainer. She is living a life she could never have dreamed would be possible. Her life is in balance and she's leading the life God has always intended her to live.

You see, losing weight is not the real answer to our problems. But being overweight is often the warning sign that we are not where we need to be in life.

The real answer is that we need to live a balanced life.

If you just want to work a weight-loss program, go ahead and try a couple. There are a lot of them out there. What this book and the First Place 4 Health program is all about is so much more than weight loss.

God wants to deal with all aspects of your life—the mental, the emotional, the spiritual and the physical. He wants to bring all four areas into balance. He desires to change you and me for the better by altering the way we think, the way we feel, the way we act and the way we approach life. This kind of change takes time, which is the primary reason that First Place 4 Health is different from other weight-loss programs.

This total-health program is not just about helping you lose weight. It's about helping you make the best choices to ensure that the positive changes you do make last your whole life.

Just Give Us a Year

In this book you will learn what a balanced life looks like. In the pages to come, you will find the key to permanent positive change in each of the four main components of life—the spiritual, the mental, the physical and the emotional—and discover how to find balance in each area.

When you start practicing the disciplines that bring balance, it's okay not to do every suggestion right away. This is a journey—your journey. And it will take awhile to get to the destination. Real change always takes time. This book is about making a decision to do whatever is the next right thing that will lead to positive change. Start there. Make that choice. Maybe you will begin by walking for just a few minutes a day. Maybe at first you'll just walk out to the mailbox and back. Even that amount of movement will generate some change. Your body will start to move toward a balance that it perhaps has not known in a long time.

I wish I could say that I've fully arrived after 27 years of learning how to live a balanced life. But everything in us resists change when we've done things a certain way for many years. Our minds resist a new way of thinking and our bodies rebel at changing the way we eat and the way we move. The apostle Paul talks about a similar struggle in Romans 7—he says that the things he wants to do, he often doesn't do;

and the things he doesn't want to do, he finds himself doing (see v. 19)! I often find myself in that place too.

I remember one time not too long ago when I brought some work home that I needed to do before the next day. My husband, Johnny, was not feeling well and I was in a bit of a funk myself. Although I don't watch much television, I relax by doing Sudoku puzzles—one right after another, for hours at a time. I completely avoided doing the next right thing, which was the work I had brought home, and instead escaped in doing the Sudoku puzzles. I'm not saying that God disapproves of doing Sudoku puzzles, but He had something better for me, and I chose to ignore His plan. When I decided to stop escaping, I was faced with the fact that my work was still there and now I had to sacrifice what I could have been doing—spending time on the pier, looking at the water with my precious husband—to do the work that could no longer be ignored.

Learning to give Christ first place in your life includes learning new ways to think, new ways to feel and new ways to act. These kinds of changes are what will make permanent lifestyle changes possible. These changes may not happen quickly, but they will happen, if you don't give up.

If First Place 4 Health were just a weight-loss program, there's a good chance that nothing would ever truly change in your life. But here's my promise to you: *Give God and First Place 4 Health one year . . . and your life will change forever.*

Do some math with me. At First Place 4 Health, we never encourage anyone to lose more than two pounds a week. Just two pounds. Sometimes success can be measured in not losing any weight at all. Rather, success might lie in not gaining weight. For some people, the biggest problem is how to stop gaining.

Think of it this way. For several years now, the number of gastric bypass surgeries—stomach stapling, lap band, or the more invasive permanent reduction of the stomach—has grown astronomically throughout North America. Practitioners promise that you will lose 100 pounds in a year. I have a friend who had gastric bypass surgery. She did lose 130 pounds the first year, but she has gained back 50 pounds since then. Here's the problem: Surgery does nothing to change the issues that brought about the weight gain in the first place. Surgery addresses only the physical. It's an imbalanced solution. Besides that, surgery is expensive, it complicates your lifestyle and it's risky; people have been known to die from it.

We have several leaders who have had gastric bypass surgery and they realize they still must live the First Place 4 Health lifestyle to keep their life in balance. If you have had weight-loss surgery, First Place 4 Health will help you learn how to bring balance to every area of your life.

Following the First Place 4 Health program, if you lose just 2 pounds a week, you'll lose 104 pounds in a year. You will have lost the same amount of weight you would have lost with gastric bypass surgery, but your life will be totally different from the way it would have been with the surgery.

So give us one year, and allow God to work the way He wants to work in your life. It's not just about losing weight; it's about making lifestyle changes that affect your body, soul, mind and emotions.

True, First Place 4 Health does teach you how to deal with your weight—but that's a side benefit. At its core, First Place 4 Health teaches you how to deal with life.

Here's my other promise to you: *First Place 4 Health is not a diet.*

Anyone who has ever struggled with weight gain knows what a diet is. It means endless small plates of chicken breast, and salad without dressing.

What a wonderful world we live in with all the varieties of food God gives us—the most succulent tomatoes, the juiciest squash, the perfect strawberry, the hearty loaf of whole grain bread.

We want to show you how to eat—and eat well. This is not an invitation to gluttony. It's an invitation to health. Let me stress that First Place is not a *diet*. First Place is a *live-it*. In the pages to come, you will learn how to truly live.

Your Plan for Making Positive Choices

Maybe a lifestyle change is more than some of you want—*Just help me take off the pounds,* you say.

I understand that. When I joined First Place in March 1981, the only change I desired was to lose weight. I had lost weight many times before, but I always gained it back. I saw First Place as just one more weight-loss program, with the added spiritual twist of giving Christ first place. Looking back, I admit that I didn't have a clue about what it meant to give Christ first place in everything, because I had always occupied that position!

My life today is living proof of what Christ can do when He's given the opportunity to make changes His way and in His time. My First Place 4 Health journey has been about learning how to let Christ change me from the inside out, one small change at a time. Has it been easy? No. Has it been worth it? Absolutely! No dollar value can be placed on the changes Christ has made in my life. My only regret is that I didn't start sooner.

Change is a given that can either be for our harm or for our good.

Your specific choice today is whether or not to say yes to positive change.

Are you willing? Or if that's going too fast, are you willing to let God show you what it means to be willing?

Today can be the beginning of a brand-new life. When you walk down this road, you're going to find out who God is and how wonderful He is. His desire is to make you into the person He has destined you to be from the day you were born. And I guarantee that you'll want to find out who He created you to be! God always has something so much better for us than we could ever imagine: namely, the abundant life He has promised for those who follow Him.

Are you willing to join me on this exciting journey of change? I promise that if you don't quit, you will succeed. Success is found in the process. Permanent success and lifestyle changes do not happen quickly, but they do happen if you continue to walk consistently in the same positive direction. So give us just one year. By then you will have lost the weight you want to lose or be well on your way to your goal. You will also have begun to experience the balanced life you have always desired, finding health, healing and wholeness along the way.

Chapter 1

Get on the Bus

One of my favorite authors and speakers, Patsy Clairmont, tells the story of when her son was about six years old. Because they lived out in the country, she walked her son to the bus stop every morning. One day, early in the school year, before she got back to the house, she heard the footsteps of her son running up behind her.

"What in the world are you doing?" she said to him. "The school bus will be here any minute."

"I'm quitting school," he said, looking her straight in the eye.

"You can't quit school," she replied. "You're only in first grade. Why do you want to quit?"

"Well, it's too long, too hard and too boring," he said.

"Son, that's life," said Patsy. "Get on the bus."

* * *

Have you ever wanted to give up?

There's a worthy goal ahead, but to reach the goal takes time, effort and focus. When you run into obstacles, your first inclination might be to quit. That's when the best thing you can do is square your shoulders, set your lunch kit firmly under your arm and get on the bus—in other words, take one simple step toward your goal.

If you're reading this book, chances are good that you have a worthy goal in mind—you want your life and health to change for the better.

Maybe you haven't fully articulated the goal, but you know that you can't stay the same. You know that something has to change in your life because parts of your life—perhaps *all* parts—aren't what they could be right now.

What's the most obvious part of your life that needs to change—is it your weight?

Being overweight is an obvious catalyst that invites you to open the door to positive change. It's easy to admit to a struggle with weight when the mirrors, the scale and the clothes closets in your house don't lie. Being overweight is noticeable—to you and to others. You can't ignore it. It never lets you forget its presence.

- *Maybe you feel the extra weight in your heart and lungs.* It's difficult to climb stairs. It's difficult or impossible to play with your kids or grandchildren. You dread your annual physical checkup because you already know what the doctor is going to tell you.

- *Perhaps buying clothes is distressing and embarrassing for you.* You see the clothes you'd like to wear, but nothing fits or feels right. You dread wearing shorts. You detest wearing a swimsuit, and you might even refuse to participate in any activity that requires your wearing a swimsuit.

- *Maybe you sense a subtle discrimination at work.* You are passed over for a promotion and wonder if it has anything to do with your weight. Maybe your sales would be higher if you looked fit. Maybe you'd get more respect if you weren't packing on the pounds.

- *You dread social events, such as a class reunion, where you're with people who haven't seen you for a while.* You hear people say good things to others, but no positive comments come your way. Maybe people give you pointed stares. Maybe they even joke that your spouse's cooking must be really good.

• *Weight affects your pocketbook.* Your grocery bill is higher. Your life insurance premiums are elevated. You spend more on medical deductibles. Maybe you have paid a lot of money for weight-loss programs and related books.

• *You fear the severe repercussions of being overweight.* One of your grandmothers suffers from diabetes. An uncle died of heart disease. Another had a stroke. You're about the same age and condition as they were when their bodies became diseased. What will be your fate?

The reasons why you are overweight are numerous. You may have struggled with weight forever. You've always been the "fat kid," the one picked last in gym class, the girl without a date at prom or the tubby guy who's always good for a joke. You blame the weight on your genes, the way you were raised or the fact that your mother always cooked with butter. But it doesn't matter—in the end you're overweight because you've always been that way.

Some people struggle with weight only after a major life change—the pounds came on after marriage, after reaching a certain age, during pregnancy. You remember what it was like to be fit, but that was definitely yesterday's body. You see pictures of yourself taken a few years ago, before you gained weight, and wonder if you'll ever look like that again.

Some of us wrestle with weight because, in our most honest moments, we know it acts as a cocoon. If this is your reason, perhaps you gained weight because something terrible happened years ago. Maybe your father died when you were young and you're still grieving his loss;

you were date raped as a teenager and it has taken years to overcome the tragedy; you went through an ugly divorce and are still scarred and wounded. The extra pounds feel like a protection. You believe your weight hides you from a hurtful world. Food is a refuge that always seems to make you feel better.

Some people struggle with weight because age or other health conditions hinder ease of movement. If this is your story, you long to be fit and healthy, but most mornings when you wake up you simply feel miserable. It's hard to get off the couch, much less walk around the block.

Others struggle with weight because life moves too fast. You've got to work all day and pick up the kids after soccer practice and get dinner on the table and make phone calls for the committee after dinner and on and on and on—how can you possibly take time to focus on your health?

Whatever the reasons, you know one thing for sure: The pounds are there, and you wish they weren't. You long for a better life—a vibrant, healthy life. Deep down you long to be the kind of person whose life is characterized by balance and satisfaction.

You can glimpse the better goal of being fit and well, but to reach that goal, you know it will take time, effort and focus. Obstacles will come up—they've come up every other time you've tried to lose weight, and when this happens, the temptation is always to quit. You know that you need to take one simple step at a time toward your target. But how do you do that?

The Place to Begin

There is hope for your future weight loss, and it's found in a place you may have never imagined. The easy thing would be for me to give you another diet to follow. But statistics tell us that 95 percent of people who lose weight gain it back again.[1] The simple fact is that another diet is not the solution you're looking for.

I repeat: If all you're looking for is a quick way to lose weight, then this book will disappoint you. That's not what First Place 4 Health is all about. Besides, I won't give you a quick fix that will take the pounds off only to have them come back on a short time later.

I want to give you a lasting solution that addresses not only the number you see on a scale but also your whole person—spiritually, mentally, emotionally and physically. It's the plan that helps you lead the life you were meant to live—a good life filled with hope, purpose and health.

If that kind of life is something that interests you, I want to let you in on a little secret. The hope for your future weight loss begins with this simple fact:

God is good.

That's where the First Place 4 Health program begins. Does that statement sound so simple that you feel like dismissing it? "God is good" is one of the most far-reaching principles of the Bible, and it affects your life in ways that you may never have imagined. Let's take that one fact and unpack it a bit.

Imagine for a moment that you lived a few thousand years ago. You're in a community of people loved by God, but you have all made mistakes over a long period of time, and you find yourself conquered, captured and carted off to Babylon by order of King Nebuchadnezzar.

In this new land, nothing feels the same and nothing looks the same. Obstacles are all around you. You're a stranger in a strange land. But you get a letter from one of your "pastors"—the prophet Jeremiah—and the letter lays out the very words of God.

In the letter, God says that He knows everything there is to know about you, including the events of your life that have led you to this place of exile. God knows the mistakes you have made, but He offers you His grace. The Lord declares these simple yet profound words:

I know the plans I have for you, plans to prosper you and not
to harm you, plans to give you hope and a future (Jer. 29:11).

That's the simple fact: God has good plans for you, plans to give you a
hope and a future. In other words—God is good.

God is the same yesterday, today and tomorrow. Even though He
wrote those words through the prophet Jeremiah, to a specific group of
people at a specific place and time, His righteous character is still the
same toward us today. Whenever we turn to the Lord and ask for His
help, He extends His hand of grace to us.

Nahum 1:7 repeats that thought:

The Lord is good, a refuge in times of trouble.
He cares for those who trust in Him.

That's the real answer to your goal of losing weight and becoming
healthy. Start with the fact that *God is good*. He cares for you. The answer
you're looking for encompasses not just taking off pounds, but also living the life of purpose and hope you were meant to live. This is the life
God calls you to live. And that life is well within your grasp. This book
will show you what it's all about.

Do the Next Right Thing

To begin learning about this new, healthier lifestyle, you need to start
right where you are. That means taking whatever positive step is right
in front of you; or, in other words, "do the next right thing."

I want to share with you part of a letter I received from one of our
First Place 4 Health group leaders. She has chosen to show up to life every
day. She takes small steps. She makes ordinary decisions for positive
change. But she is walking the path of balance that leads to total health.

I have battled depression most of my life. When I became a Christian, that battle did not go away. In 1990, when I weighed 220 pounds, I prayed that God would deliver me from my addiction to food. One week later, I learned about First Place. (First Place has been a lifesaver for me. I have been a First Place leader off and on since 1991.)

When my mother came to live with us, and I became her full-time caregiver, I dropped out of First Place and my weight went up to 273 pounds. I am disabled and live with chronic pain on a daily basis. During this time there were days when I only got out of bed to take care of my mother's most basic needs.

When she went home to be with the Lord in 2002, I chose to have gastric bypass surgery the next year instead of returning to First Place. I lost 90 pounds the first year and then stopped. I have since realized that there's no magic cure for weight gain. Even with gastric bypass surgery, the answer is to eat less and exercise more.

I wanted so badly to start leading First Place again, but since I'd had weight-loss surgery, I felt that I couldn't justify leading the class. I prayed and sought the Lord and called your office and was encouraged to share with the class and go forward. I have done that now for the last two years.

All of this leads up to why I am writing. I have battled depression since I was a very young girl. God has helped me so much since becoming a Christian, but it is a battle every day, and some days I lose the fight. One of my First Place assistants brought a copy of the April 2007 First Place Newsletter to class for each of our members. That newsletter has changed my life.

We all have Aha! moments in life when one word or one Scripture reaches us and the light bulb turns on. For me it was one line from that newsletter. "When there are times when all I

can do is the next right thing, then I do the next right thing."
Wow! I thought. *Maybe I can do that.* So I typed up this saying
and placed it on my bathroom mirror. The very next day I woke
up in great pain, not knowing how to begin doing all the things
I needed to do, and with no energy and no desire to do anything. Then I remembered the saying—*Do the next right thing.*
I read it out loud, and I read it again. And then, I did the next
right thing. All day that day, if I got confused or overwhelmed
or sad, I went back to the bathroom and read that statement
and then did the next right thing.

My husband can't believe the things I have gotten accomplished. My house is cleaner; my laundry is done (folded *and*
put away); I go to bed earlier and get up earlier. I have started
swimming at the YWCA. I have become interested in reading
and doing crafts again. Previously, I just wanted to stay in bed
until noon; but now I tell myself to just get up and do the next
right thing.

The words "Do the next right thing" have completely
changed my life. Do I still battle depression? Yes. Maybe I will
for the rest of my life unless the Lord chooses to heal me. Am I
still in constant pain? Oh, yes. I need surgery, and maybe now
I will find the courage to go ahead with that. But I don't have
to worry about that—I just have to do the next right thing.

In the pages ahead, you will see more specifically what taking positive steps looks like. Together we will examine the model of the four-
sided person and explore what it means to live a balanced life mentally,
spiritually, emotionally and physically. You are invited to make foundational shifts toward positive habits that will help you along your new
journey. Through the power of God, you can decide to live a healthier
life, and you can experience lasting positive change.

When I think of a person who has succeeded in this area, I think of my friend Deborah, a woman in my First Place 4 Health group.

Deborah had a number of strikes against her. At 5'8", she weighed more than 200 pounds. She had been in an emotionally and physically abusive marriage and was in the process of getting a divorce. She had custody of her two preteen girls and was tired a lot. After suffering from chronic depression for years, Deborah was on several medications.

When Deborah came to her first meeting, all she did was sit. She sat through an entire 12-week session and didn't lose a pound.

She signed up for another 12-week session. She came and sat, and didn't lose a pound.

So she signed up for a third 12-week session. On the day the session was to start, she sent me this email: "Carole, please take my name off the roll. I'm just dragging the group down."

I knew that Deborah wasn't doing her Bible study. I knew that she had not learned the food plan. I knew that she was convinced that all she was able to do was sit. And I knew that she had reached the point where the pain of not changing was forcing her to move beyond the lies and make a choice. Her choice was that she needed to *make a choice*.

I replied to her email message with one line: *Deborah—just come today.*

That day, when Deborah arrived, I hugged her, and she started crying.

That was her moment of choice. From that moment on, she started responding to the program. She began doing her Bible study and memorizing verses. She started walking around her neighborhood with her girls. She started eating according to the Live It plan.

Soon, she had lost 60 pounds.

Previously hidden aspects of Deborah's personality began to shine through. She was fun! We learned that she was a talented photographer. In fact, in March 2006, she went to Israel with a tour group arranged by First Place 4 Health. She took pictures for the group and walked up and down the rocky terrain. I had never seen her like that—so vibrant and full of action. She had just been so squashed down all of her life.

"Deborah," I said, a while ago, "tell me what finally happened for you to make a choice."

"Carole," she said, "you believed in me. You believed that I could do it. Nobody ever believed in me before."

What she said is true. I believed in her. And I believe in you. I believe that you can do it. Even if no one has ever believed in you before, know that someone believes in you now. With God's help, you can change. It's your choice. And you have the power to do it.

As you take your next steps toward positive change, keep in mind that you must choose to change before change will begin.

First Place 4 Health is not a diet; it's a lifestyle shift.

People often believe that if they can just get on the right diet, all their weight problems will be solved. That's an easy mistake to make, because the latest, greatest diets are always marketed as the solution we need. Yet First Place 4 Health is much more than a diet; it's a change in how to approach life. The good thing about the First Place 4 Health food plan is that it's not restrictive like a diet would be. We invite you to explore all the wonderful world of food choices the Lord has provided.

- *First Place 4 Health is not about rigid rules; it's about helpful invitations.* We used to stress *commitments*—which is a good concept. We wanted people to be dedicated to pursuing health. But we have found that people sometimes looked at commitments as laws, and if laws were broken, then guilt and rigidity set in. Instead, we are inviting you to make a number of positive changes in your life. No one does them all perfectly, all of the time. So relax. There isn't just one way to live a healthy life. Develop the plan that works best for you, and give yourself grace to make mistakes and adjustments along the way.

• *Get involved at your own pace.* When it comes to living a healthy, balanced life, success will look different for different people. Some people lose 100 pounds the first year they're involved in First Place 4 Health. Other people lose 20 pounds and keep it off for 20 years. For others, success is found in *not gaining* any more weight. You are welcome in First Place 4 Health regardless of where you are with your current level of health. We encourage you to do no more than what you are ready for. Yet we do encourage you to take a first positive step as soon as possible.

• *Your invitation starts right now.* Any change requires some sort of adjustment. Your invitation is to jump in to this new life today. Just begin. Get on the bus. Make the choice to give yourself wholeheartedly to this new season in your life—a season that will hopefully stretch into a lifetime of healthy living. Have fun exploring new ways to grow in your faith and in your understanding of health. Develop new friendships by getting involved in something good for you. Don't be satisfied with standing on the outside—come on in! Be courageous and take the next step in living a balanced life.

What Keeps You Going?

The formula for lasting change:

A worthy goal reached through time + effort + focus

When obstacles to meeting your goal come up, your first inclination may be to quit. That's when you take the next step toward your goal— just one simple step at a time.

It helps to have a clear idea of what a worthy goal looks like. You may not have articulated more than the words "to lose weight." While this is a worthy goal, it usually breaks down when obstacles come up, because you need a greater understanding of the motivation behind your goal. When you remember why it is that you wanted to lose weight in the first place, that knowledge keeps you heading toward your goal.

People lose weight for all sorts of reasons. The Bible provides the foundational motivation, and it's as simple as this: God is interested in your health. The motivations are shown in two passages of Scripture. Check out Romans 12:1-2:

> Therefore, I urge you, brothers, in view of God's mercy, to offer your bodies as living sacrifices, holy and pleasing to God—this is your spiritual act of worship. Do not conform any longer to the pattern of this world, but be transformed by the renewing of your mind. Then you will be able to test and approve what God's will is—his good, pleasing and perfect will.

In other words, you are urged to present your body—your actual flesh and blood and bone and skin—to God as an act of worship. How you take care of your body is a reflection of what you think about God. It's honoring to the Lord to take care of the body He has given you.

When your body is presented to God, He invites you to use your life in service to Him.

> Do you not know that your body is a temple of the Holy Spirit, who is in you, whom you have received from God? You are not your own; you were bought at a price. Therefore honor God with your body (1 Cor. 6:19-20).

The benefit here is yours. To live for the Lord God of All is an incredible privilege. God's invitation is to an abundant life full of purpose and hope. A foundational motivation for weight loss and total lifestyle change is to give your body to God.

It seems strange to think about it, but if you have accepted Christ as your Savior, then you have the actual Spirit of God living inside your body. It doesn't make you a god. It means that your body houses the spirit of God, and that He works in your life by faith.

So what are the foundational motivations for losing weight and living a life of balance?

First, *God wants you to.* God is interested in your health.

Second, when your life is in balance, it's much easier to be a leader in your family and a role model for your children and spouse. It's difficult to lead people where you have never been yourself. Many children are overweight and need encouragement from their parents. Many of the weight problems of our children would evaporate if we led by example.

I've experienced this truth in my own life. When I first started to exercise, my oldest granddaughter, Cara, loved to walk or jog with me. Would she have done it on her own? No way! Yet in a heartbeat, she came with me at my invitation. Children love being with their family members.

Third, weight loss can also expose the true needs in our hearts. I'm talking specifically to those of you who need emotional healing. A weight gain is often a symptom of a deeper issue. For instance, women and men who have been emotionally or sexually abused often attempt to hide their pain by eating.

But whatever motivation is speaking to your heart, just take a moment now to get on the bus.

In the space on the following pages, jot down some ideas about the reasons you want to lose weight. It can be very beneficial to see your goals on paper. When obstacles come (and they will), you can refer back to this to gain encouragement.

Sometimes it helps to record a positive goal as well as its negative extrapolation of what might happen if you don't do anything. Sometimes it can help to imagine your life in 5, 10 or 15 years. What will happen if something changes? What will happen if nothing changes?

Take some time to think through the following declarations.

I want to lose weight because . . .

_____

_____

_____

_____

_____

I want to lose weight so that I can . . .

_____

_____

_____

_____

and be a good example to . . .

_____

_____

_____

_____

If I lose weight, then in the future I can see myself . . .

_____

_____

_____

_____

If I don't lose weight, then in the future I can see myself . . .

_____

_____

_____

_____

There is no correct way to word your goal. What matters is that you know your goal, remind yourself of it often and keep in mind that your goal is reachable. With God's help, you can do it.

Congratulations! You're on Your Way

God never promised us that life would be rosy and without difficulty. Instead, the Lord promises to carry us through any situation and trial. God already knows your goals. He knows that you desire a better life filled with purpose, health and hope. And He knows the obstacles you will encounter that tempt you to quit the journey. Don't give up! You can make it!

Remember, you have already taken the first step by reading this chapter. And it wasn't that hard. Now you're on the bus! You're on your way to a whole new you.

Checklist for Success

- Acknowledge the truth that God is good and that He offers you a hope-filled plan for your life and future. Your success begins with this simple fact.

- Run from quick fixes—they never provide you with the lasting change you need. First Place 4 Health is a lifestyle change that affects your whole person—mentally, spiritually, emotionally, physically. It will take time, but it's worth it.

• Accept the invitation to give your life to God. He is interested in everything about you—including your physical health.

• Write down the specific reasons why you want to become healthy. Refer back to your declarations often for motivation. Remind yourself why not doing anything isn't an option.

• Start today. Obstacles and excuses will come up, but quitting isn't the answer. *Do the next right thing!*

Note
1. This statistic is frequently cited in weight-loss journals and health-related articles, for example: http://preventdisease.com/fitness/weightloss/articles/carbs.html (accessed January 23, 2007).

Chapter 2

Never Diet Again

Before I joined the First Place 4 Health program in 1981, I had been on lots of diets. You see, although I was only 20 pounds overweight, it looked like much more on my 5'3" frame.

By the time I was 40, I was quite familiar with those 20 pounds. When they showed up at my door every year during the holiday season, I'd beat them away with whatever diet was current. Maybe the pounds would show up again during the year in a season of stress, and I'd beat them away again. But they never left for good. The same 20 pounds came back again and again.

The problem with any diet I tried is that my motivation was misguided. In the end, the real reasons why I gained weight were still there. The diet never addressed why I put on those extra pounds in the first place. Sure, I lost weight on diets—maybe there was a reunion I needed to attend or a wedding where I knew a lot of photos would be taken. Diet time! Got to get that weight down for the big event. But as soon as the wedding was over, it was the same old me eating the same old way I had always eaten.

Of all the misguided motivations to lose weight, I think one of the worst is when a spouse dangles a financial carrot. A husband might look at his wife and say, "Honey, if you lose 50 pounds, you can spend $500 on a new wardrobe."

The thought of shopping for cute new clothes can be enticing, but the destructive, not-so-subtle message is: "You're not okay as you are.

You would look a whole lot better if you weren't so fat. In fact, I'll pay for you to get slim."

If you're motivated to lose weight only to please someone else—a spouse, a parent, a friend—what happens when problems arise or the relationship changes? What happens when all of those cute new clothes get old? Chances are, you will return to eating the way you've always eaten.

If you want true, lasting weight loss, you've got to address more than the surface issue of shedding pounds. First Place 4 Health's primary goal is not to change the numbers on the scale. We want to show you how to live a balanced life—mentally, physically, emotionally, and spiritually. When your life is in balance, you will also achieve lasting weight loss.

Throughout this book you will learn more about what living a balanced life looks like; but first, take a look at why you are overweight in the first place. By examining these issues, you will finally shed some light on the real reasons you are overweight and begin your journey toward a healthy lifestyle.

A Series of Small, Positive Choices

It can be scary to think of lifting the lid to your inner life. It's much safer to keep things the way they are. We don't want to do any work; we want quick fixes. "Oh, if only there were a magic pill that would make all this weight go away," we say with a sigh.

Here's a cold, hard fact: *There is no magic pill.* There is no quick fix. Think of it this way: How long did it take to get to the place you are today? Being unhealthy doesn't happen overnight. As strange as it sounds, the patterns and habits that lead to feeling miserable take a long time to become ingrained in your system.

Here's another fact: You didn't get unhealthy overnight and you won't get healthy overnight either.

Please don't let that statement get you down. Knowing the true characteristics of any battle is part of the successful strategy we must employ to win it. We are in this battle together, and patience is part of the plan for victory.

People of faith often look for a quick solution; we long for a miracle. We think, *If only Jesus would come through and instantly make me well.*

Sometimes the Lord, in His grace, does it this way. But instant divine healings are the exception, not the norm. God wants us to use all the faculties we've been given. He is interested in our healing, but He wants us to use our wisdom, knowledge and skills too.

In fact, God is always respectful of our right to choose—whether we choose a healthy lifestyle or an unhealthy one. He is the perfect gentleman. He doesn't crowd His way into our lives. He lets us make decisions for our harm as well as our good.

What we often long for is to be super-Christians. We wish that we instantly knew all the answers to life's dilemmas. We wish that we always did the right thing. We wish that we never had to learn anything—that we automatically possessed all the wisdom there is.

Let me give you a third fact: *There is no such thing as a super-Christian.*

We all have to learn things along the way. We all make mistakes. We're all sinners and fall short of the glory of God (see Rom. 3:23). We're all on a learning curve during life's journey.

One of the core tenets of the First Place 4 Health program is that we're all people in process. What leads to lasting success is making a series of small, positive choices every day.

A friend of mine was struggling with an issue with her mother. The friend had spent the day at her mother's house and had come home in tears to her husband. The mother was going through a rough time herself, and the daughter was grieving the rough time, but she also felt that her mother was acting overly needy and clingy. She wasn't experiencing the friendship she had always hoped she would have with her mother. Relationships between adult women and their mothers can be complex things!

There would be no solution that night. No quick fix. No easy answer. No super-Christian thing to do. Success for my friend was simply found in going to bed that night and getting enough sleep. (One small decision.) The next morning she got up and took care of her family—getting her two young daughters up, bathed, fed and off to preschool and first grade. (More small decisions.) She then took care of herself—making sure that she ate well and went to aerobics and came home and had a shower and got dressed and read her Bible and prayed and wrote a short note to her mother to encourage her. (Small decisions, all of them.)

Soon my friend came to realize that perhaps the larger problem would never get totally solved. Life can often be that way. Human relationships are seldom tidy. But what led her to lasting success was a series of small, positive choices, day after day after day.

Why Are We Overweight?

We can have that kind of success, too, but first we need to look at some of the reasons why we are overweight to begin with. By examining these issues, we'll begin to see the real reasons why we live the way we do now. Then we can start the real work of progressing on this journey toward total health.

The problems include hiding, being fearful and running away.

We Hide

Our natural tendency is to hide from self, from other healthy relationships and from God.

Hiding is one of the core patterns of human behavior seen in the Bible. After Adam and Eve sinned in the Garden of Eden, they realized their nakedness for the first time as mistrust and alienation set in.

What was the first thing they did?

They covered themselves with fig leaves.

In other words—they hid.

This is a tendency we all have. When we make mistakes or dabble in sin or have something bad happen to us, we don't want to call attention to what's wrong. We don't want to call truth what it is. We'd much rather quietly explain away the unhealthiness. Any excuse we make really means that we'd rather hide the truth.

Hiding can take a lot of forms. We hide whenever we whisper things to ourselves such as:

- No one will see me eat this half-gallon of ice cream tonight all by myself.

- I hate the thought of meeting with other people for help and advice. I'd much rather just try to get healthy on my own.

- I've just sinned, and I'm ashamed of it, but I surely can't face God now. I hate the thought of praying for help. God doesn't want anything to do with me. I'd rather eat than turn to God.

Do some hard work right now and take a look inward. When you examine your inner life, is there anything you're hiding from? If so, have the courage to write down one line that identifies what you're hiding from. You take a very large step toward health when you get your hidden issue out in the open.

When I'm absolutely honest with myself, I have to admit that I'm hiding from . . .

_____

_____

_____

We Fear

We fear what we can't control. We fear what might happen. We fear being judged by others. We fear who we think God is and what He thinks of us.

Fear can be a hugely debilitating presence in our life. Fear keeps us from doing what we know is right. Fear insists that we can't make positive choices, or we don't have the power to do anything about the situation we're in. Fear keeps us inside our houses and isolated from other people. Fear keeps us from opening our Bibles and makes us turn away from God when we're in need.

Fear can also take a lot of forms. Fear shows up anytime we whisper things like:

- I'm alone, I've always been alone, I can't handle being alone. I'm going to eat something to make me feel better.

- People hate me. They look down on me. No one knows what I'm going through. It's safer to eat than talk.

- I have to perform. I can't let people down. If other people are disappointed in me, that would be horrible. Eating helps keep me safe.

- God has no idea what I'm going through and He doesn't care. Since God can't understand me, I'm afraid of His reaction whenever I do something that I know is unhealthy.

When you truly examine your inner life, is there anything you're fearful of? Do some core work and have the courage to write down at least one of your fears. Getting it out in the open can be a very healthy step to take.

When I'm absolutely honest with myself, I have to admit that I fear . . .

_____

_____

_____

_____

We Run

We tend to run toward quick fixes—toward unhealthy activities, substances or practices that we believe will help us. We run away from healthy friendships. And we run away from God.

Running is a natural tendency whenever we encounter something that's hard to handle. Running is instinctive—we want to get away from something that is hurtful or difficult, and we want to run toward something that we think will be helpful, even when it's not.

We run anytime we say things like:

- I can't handle life right now. Food will make me feel better. Eating always makes me feel better.

- I need to lose weight fast—I'm going to try that 10 pounds in 10 days diet I heard about on TV.

- My friend invited me out for coffee, but I don't think I'll go. She always asks me hard questions.

- God doesn't care about me. I want to stay as far away from Him as I can.

The small positive step of writing things down is important. Secrets flourish in the dark. Truth needs light. Have the courage to write down one thing you're running from—get it out in the open.

When I'm absolutely honest with myself, I know I'm running from ... (or toward ...)

_____

_____

_____

Looking at some of your core motivations for overeating is never easy. In fact, the issues in your life may be far more complex than what you can adequately express in a few lines. It's okay to continue doing more core work on your own. People have been known to fill up whole journals just by asking themselves the basic questions: What am I hiding from? What do I fear? What am I running from?

Getting a handle on your motivations for overeating is key. But you don't want to leave it there. Scripture reveals a much more hopeful path by bringing important truths into our lives—truths that will change our way of thinking and our way of living.

Help for Today

The solution to our desire to lose weight is not that we go on another diet; the solution is to make a lifestyle change. Lasting change happens when we make a series of small, positive choices day after day.

What are the truths that will help you along this journey? Let's look at several of them together.

The truth is mapped throughout Scripture, but one passage stands out boldly on this subject. It's found in Hebrews 4:13-16. From these verses we learn that the truth is . . .

God knows everything, so we don't need to hide.

He knows everything there is to know about everything—including everything about you. If that sounds scary, it doesn't need to be.

Remember the foundational truth we talked about in the last chapter? *God is good.* So couple what you know of God's good character with His knowledge of you.

Hebrews 4:13 says:

> Nothing in all creation is hidden from God's sight. Everything is uncovered and laid bare before the eyes of Him to whom we must give account.

If God knows everything (and He is good), then you don't have to hide anything from Him. In fact, you *can't* hide anything from God.

The phrase "we must give account" can sound ominous. Scripturally, this refers to a gain or loss of reward someday when we all stand before Christ. But again, God is a good God. The emphasis of this verse isn't that God is going to whack us over the head with a two-by-four but that He is very much aware of all that is going on in our life.

Armed with this fact, Scripture encourages us not to hide. Hiding is futile. The opposite of hiding is being known. That's both a comforting and a sobering fact.

What might this scriptural truth look like in your life?

- If you ever try to eat a half-gallon of ice cream in secret, know that you're in God's presence. God loves you and is always there to help you.

- Meeting other trusted friends for help and encouragement is a good thing. It's virtually impossible to become healthy on your own. The time for living in secret is over.

- Whenever you sin, and shame takes hold of your life, you're still in God's presence. God knows the sin but reaches out to you always. Just like the father who welcomed his prodigal son with open arms (see Luke 15:11-31), God always welcomes you home.

Take a moment to write down something about your own life that will help you remember this truth. God knows everything, so you don't need to hide. What might that look like in your life?

Since God knows everything, and I don't have to hide anymore, that means . . .

_____

_____

_____

_____

_____

Here's the second truth:

God is sympathetic, so we don't have to fear.

God is full of compassion. He deals gently with us. He knows what it's like to be a human being. He sent His Son, Jesus Christ, to Earth, where Jesus was tempted in every way known to mankind without giving in to those temptations. That's what makes Him our Savior and Redeemer. It also makes Him full of compassion for all the ways we are tempted to fall.

People who follow Christ can exhibit the same compassion. Maybe you've been hurt by others in the past and your guard is up; but not everybody is like that. Yes, we're all sinners, but not everyone is cruel, hateful or mean.

The First Place 4 Health program offers the supportive community of small groups to help you along your way. The people in these groups aren't perfect, but all who attend are committed to support-ing and encouraging their fellow group members. It's a built-in sup-port network.

A woman in my First Place 4 Health group, Dee, encountered this support firsthand.

Dee had spent much of her life, in her own words, "trying to fly under the radar." Her goal was to not attract any attention to herself. Imbalance had led to weight issues, and her health was always a concern. She had been on her own since she was a young teenager and frequently experienced fear of abandonment. She had three children—a 19-year-old, a 12-year-old and a 6-year-old. Like a lot of parents, Dee worried about them constantly.

Dee seldom spoke when she first came to my group. When she did speak, she was open and transparent and offered good insights during the Bible study times. Although we wanted to hear more from her, her comments were few.

You would hardly recognize the old Dee today. She has experi-enced such emotional healing that she is now co-leader of a group. She has learned to trust God and to pray. And she is on her way to her weight goal.

I asked Dee some time ago when the change happened.

"People just didn't let me fly under the radar," she said. "So I made a simple choice to commit to being there—even if I'd had a rotten week. I just decided to always show up—I knew that I'd find care at the group."

That's what support and encouragement can do for you. And that's the way Jesus Christ is with you. Hebrews 4:15 describes Him:

For we do not have a high priest who is unable to sympathize with our weaknesses, but we have one who has been tempted in every way, just as we are—yet without sin.

It might seem strange to think of Jesus Christ as a high priest—it's a concept many of us aren't familiar with today. A high priest was someone who interceded for people—a spiritual leader who dealt gently with the people in his care. Christ is that to us. He understands our weaknesses.

Knowing this about Christ, we don't have to be afraid. God has compassion on us. He's not some great cosmic cop who pulls us over and takes us to jail. Armed with this fact, our fears are lessened. When there is no more fear, it's much easier to do what we know is right. Without fear, it's easier to make positive choices. Without fear, we are able to trust our friends.

When we rest secure in the knowledge that God is sympathetic to us, we can say things like:

- I'm never alone. A good God is always with me. I don't need to eat something to make me feel better; I can turn to Him. He knows what I'm feeling right now.

- People don't hate me or look down on me. Others know what I'm going through. I have a trusted group of friends—I am safe with them.

- I don't have to perform. If other people are disappointed in me, it's not the end of the world. Being real and authentic is the way to live.

- God knows all about that I'm going through, and He cares. Since God understands me, I don't need to fear His reaction whenever I do something I know is unhealthy. I can always turn to Him.

Take a moment to write down something that will help you remember this truth in your life: God is sympathetic; others can be sympathetic.

What might "no fear" look like in your life?

Because God is sympathetic to me, that means I don't need to fear . . .

_____

_____

_____

_____

Here's another truth:

> *God wants to help us, so we can always approach Him.*

Perhaps the most wonderful truth of all is that God is on our side. He's for us. Because of what Christ did on the cross for us, there are no barriers to God when we ask Christ to be our Savior. We can turn to Him instead of running from Him. Hebrews 4:16 reads:

> Let us approach the throne of grace with confidence, so that we may receive mercy and find grace to help us in our time of need.

God wants to help you. Turning to God is always the solution you need. So approach Him boldly, rather than running toward the latest quick fix or the nearby doughnut shop. Remember, God is always interested in your life and always willing to help you.

Armed with this truth, you can say things like

- Life is really hard right now, but I can approach God boldly; I don't have to run to food.

- I feel like I need to lose weight fast—but I know that's not a lasting solution. So I'm not going to run to that new diet I heard about on TV; I'm going to turn to the Lord.

- My friend invited me out for coffee, and I'm going to go. She always asks me hard questions, but I don't want to run from that. I need to have close friends in my life. I'm not going to run from accountability, even though it's sometimes difficult.

- God loves me and cares about me. I can always turn to Him.

Take a moment to write down something that will help you remember the truth that you can always approach God boldly. What might that look like in your life?

Since I can approach God with confidence, that means . . .

_____

_____

_____

_____

_____

_____

Never Diet Again

First Place 4 Health is not another diet. It's a new way of seeing your life.

If you want true, lasting weight loss, you must address more than the surface issue of shedding pounds. You must take an honest look at your need to live a balanced life—mentally, physically, emotionally and spiritually.

You can choose balance! When you're living a balanced life, you will achieve lasting weight loss. And you will be well on your way to living the abundant life God intended you to live.

Checklist for Success

- First Place 4 Health is not a diet; it's a lifestyle change that addresses every aspect of your being—the mental, the spiritual, the emotional and the physical.

- Stop running to quick fixes and forget trying to be a "super-Christian." What leads to lasting success is making a series of small, positive choices day after day after day.

- It can be difficult to lift the lid on your inner life, but doing so helps you discover and address the root issues of how you got to be where you are today so that you can adjust your course.

- Weight gain happens when you hide, fear and run. Scripture offers a better path. God knows everything, so you don't need to hide. God is sympathetic, so you don't have to fear. God wants to help you, so you can always approach Him.

PART 1

Heart:
Seeking Balance Emotionally

The First Place 4 Health program is about living a balanced life—emotionally, spiritually, mentally and physically. When your life is in balance, your weight issues will be addressed in lasting ways.

Your emotions are valid, but your feelings can overtake you if you allow them. When feelings aren't based on fact, you can find yourself thinking and acting in ways that are destructive to your life and to the lives of those around you.

What does it look like to live a balanced life emotionally? That's what we'll address throughout the next two chapters.

Chapter 3

You've Gotta *Show Up*

A story is told about Martin Luther, the great sixteenth-century reformer. Although Luther's life was characterized by huge successes, he was also known for huge periods of despair.

During one such period, Luther moped around the house for days. Getting out of bed was a chore. His days were spent in blank inactivity, his nights in self-pity and moroseness.

Finally, his wife had had enough. Nothing she said seemed to be getting through to him, so she tried another tactic.

One morning she got up and dressed in her best funeral attire. Martin was shocked to see her covered from head to toe in black when she entered the kitchen that morning.

"What's the matter?" he said. "Are you going to a funeral?"

"Yes," was all she said.

"Who died?"

"God—God is dead."

"God is *not* dead!" Luther asserted.

"Well, you're sure acting like it!" his wife replied.

Luther reportedly snapped out of his despair that very morning.

I don't know how much of this story has become fictionalized over the years, and I acknowledge there are certain types of depression that require more than an attitude adjustment to overcome. But I don't want the point to be missed either.

Some of you are living as if you believe that God is dead. You're moping around the house, or you're cloaking yourself with the funeral garb of too much food, or you have convinced yourself that staying inside with the shades drawn is the safest thing you can do. You're living as if you don't believe there's a God out there who loves you and offers hope.

Luther was right—God is *not* dead! God is very much alive. God is a God of goodness and hope. He has a plan and a future for your life. He will give you the power and courage to walk this journey toward a healthy life.

But God also respects humans to such a degree that He won't make a change unless you let Him. This is about more than a one-time verbal consent. It's an attitude that is developed over time. Your invitation is to give yourself to this new attitude over the days, weeks, months and years to come—to be willing to be willing. What's the invitation?

To show up. Every day.

I'm convinced that 80 percent of life is just showing up. It means that you are ready and willing for change to take place. You have made the decision that you want to change, and you are consistently willing to take whatever steps are necessary to live this new life.

You may not do everything exactly right all of the time; but even if you get off track, whenever you *show up* you are choosing to come back to that place of balance again. When you show up, you acknowledge that God is not dead. He is alive and there is hope.

That's the first invitation—to show up day after day.

When Feelings Rule

The problem with making positive changes for our health is seldom that we don't know what to do. Usually, the challenge is to choose to do what we know to do.

You can't just sit there and do nothing. Change requires your willingness, no matter what your feelings are saying to you.

I know how hard it can be to be willing. I'm a stubborn person at heart. I began working at Houston First Baptist Church in August 1984. This is when things first began to truly change in my life in a positive way. The change was gradual, but it did happen. Even though I was already a Christian, I was shallow and weak in my faith. At heart I was a rebel, wanting to do exactly what I wanted to do whenever I wanted to do it.

My dear friend Pat Lewis (no relation, although we have the same last name), who works with me today in the offices of First Place 4 Health, also worked at the church then, and she picked me up every day and took me to work because I didn't have a car. My husband and I had recently declared bankruptcy due to a downturn in the Houston economy. Pat, who was also my co-leader in the First Place 4 Health group, was the only one who had a clue about where Johnny and I were in our personal life; and she didn't tell a soul.

Pat and I had a tradition of getting together one day every December to Christmas shop. Every year we met for breakfast and stayed together until dark. We never bought anything; we just had three meals together and talked all day. Christmas 1984 was the same as every other year. That year I was glad we didn't buy anything because I was completely broke.

At the end of the day, Pat took me home, and we sat outside my house, talking. Pat told me that God had been dealing with her during the last few weeks about something she needed to share with me. She said that she was convinced God wanted to do something great with my life and this might be my last chance—I needed to respond this time. Every sermon she had listened to at church or on the radio had screamed out to her that she had to talk to me about this issue in my life.

Pat was the only person in the world who knew what a total rebel I really was, but she loved me anyway. Her unconditional love was exactly what God used to get my attention that night. I cried, and Pat cried. I told her that I didn't know how to let go, because I felt that I had gone too far in the wrong direction. We prayed together and then parted. Little did I know this was the beginning of the unfolding of God's plan for me.

Two weeks later, on a Sunday, I was sitting in church listening to my pastor when he said something I had never heard before. He said, "God is a perfect gentleman and will not work in our life without our permission. If you are not willing, you can pray this prayer: 'Lord, I am not willing, but I am willing to be made willing.' This prayer gives God permission to begin the necessary work to help you change for the better."

As sincerely as I have ever prayed, I prayed that prayer. I told God how scared I was and that I wasn't willing, but I was willing to be made willing. I finished by asking God to not make it hurt too much. I was positive that my surrender would be a painful experience (though as it turned out, I was so wrong about that). I didn't go forward that morning during the altar call (a time during the service when the pastor invites a response of commitment from the congregation), because I worked at the church and I didn't want anyone to know what a mess I was.

The very next day, God began the work of changing me from the inside out. The most amazing thing is that even though He has changed so many of my motivations since that day, He left the person who was me intact. I still love to laugh and have fun as much as I ever did; but over the years I began to care about others more and to desire to be involved in their lives—which I honestly didn't want to do when I first joined First Place. God has used other people to help me change. He also used prayer, Bible study and Scripture memorization to bring about dramatic changes in my heart and life.

I'm sharing this part of my story because I know how difficult it can be to begin walking the road to positive change. Yet positive change cannot happen unless you make the choice to begin. *Showing up* is a metaphor for a person's willingness to do the hard work required to achieve a lifestyle change. That means you have to consciously decide to walk the journey toward living a balanced life. That decision is made more than once—it's a decision you make again and again. That's what showing up looks like: learning to begin again.

Think of it the opposite way. What does life look like when you don't show up? You back off. You take your eyes off the prize. You sneak out the back door and down the alleyway into whatever unhealthy habits are in your life.

When you don't show up, you let your feelings rule your life. You *feel* like eating an entire pizza, or you *feel* like eating a bucket of greasy chicken, or you *feel* like skipping out on your First Place 4 Health meeting for the week. The trouble with feelings is that they rule you if you let them. Why? Because the body wants to do what the body wants to do.

Feelings are funny that way. Feelings in themselves are not wrong. God gave you a full range of emotions as an expression of His righteous character. God has emotions. God expresses anger and wrath. God sorrows. God aches for lost people to come to Him. God is joyful and proud of you and tender toward you. He expresses all of His emotions in utmost righteousness.

So it's okay for you to feel your emotions. Some people say that you should only have "positive" emotions—that you should only be happy all the time, for instance. But that's not the biblical model. All that God asks of you is to be true to what He has revealed in His Word. If God calls something sinful, then He doesn't want you to be happy with sin. He wants you to be sorrowful or righteously angry toward it. If you ever find yourself wondering if a certain emotion is the accurate response to something, check it against what Scripture says.

At the same time, emotions can become a problem if you let them rule your life. That happens any time you impose a negative feeling on a situation that doesn't merit the negative emotion.

For example, it's very easy to wake up in the morning feeling grumpy and then act grumpy toward your children, your spouse or your coworkers. Why is the feeling of grumpiness there in the first place? It may have nothing to do with your children, your spouse or your coworkers, but it gets imposed on them anyway. That's when feelings become a problem.

This "the body wants to do what the body wants to do" scenario is something you must deal with. Just because your body wants sugar doesn't mean you have to give it sugar. Or just because your body wants to lie on the couch all day doesn't mean you have to give in to that desire. When your emotions prompt you to make unhealthy decisions, you have a choice to make.

Popular author and speaker Zig Ziglar describes the pathway to health as acting the way you want to feel. In other words, if you want to *feel* courageous, then *act* courageous first. This isn't being false; it's being decisive. We need to focus our minds on moving ahead—even when we don't feel like it.

Some days I don't *feel* like exercising. A thousand and one excuses crowd into my mind. If I went with my feelings, I'd just skip my workout. But regardless of my feelings, I put on my exercise clothes and step on the treadmill. I decide *to show up*. The same is true for any regular discipline, such as having my quiet time with the Lord each day or choosing to eat right. My feelings tell me to do any number of things, but balance happens when I make the decision to do the next right thing.

How about you? Take a moment to do a little inner work. Read through the list of emotions on the following page and make a note of the ones that have characterized your life in the past week or so. Then sort through the list again and note the ones you would most like your life to be characterized by. Write those emotions in the blanks below the list. (Note: There may be emotions in your life that aren't on the list. Go ahead and write those in the blanks as well.)

Accomplished	Tired	Moody	Disappointed
Aggravated	Touched	Contemplative	Discontent
Cheerful	Uncomfortable	Content	Distressed
Chipper	Anxious	Morose	Ditzy
Determined	Apathetic	Naughty	Drained
Ecstatic	Artistic	Nervous	Enraged
Sick	Awake	Nauseated	Frustrated
Creative	Blah	Grateful	Infuriated
Curious	Blank	Groggy	Indifferent
Silly	Bored	Grumpy	Irate
Sleepy	Bouncy	Guilty	Irritable
Rejuvenated	Busy	Hopeful	Jealous
Relaxed	Cold	Hungry	Jubilant
Sore	Complacent	Hyper	Lazy
Stressed	Confused	Impressed	Envious
Surprised	Pessimistic	Indescribable	Exhausted
Sympathetic	Pleased	Inefficient	Lethargic
Thankful	Passive	Happy	Listless
Thoughtful	Predatory	High	Lonely
Embarrassed	Cranky	Efficient	Nostalgic
Energetic	Crazy	Depressed	Numb
Excited	Shocked	Sad	Optimistic
Full	Crushed	Satisfied	Peaceful
Giggly	Cynical	Scared	Pensive
Giddy	Gloomy	Devious	Productive
Angry	Good	Dirty	Refreshed
Annoyed	Loved	Rejected	Stressed
Sympathetic	Melancholy	Relieved	Surprised
Thankful	Mellow	Restless	Weird
Thoughtful	Mischievous	Rushed	Worried

In the last couple of weeks, I have felt . . .

_____

_____

and _____

But I'd like to feel more . . .

_____

_____

and _____

It's okay to write *anything* in the blanks above. There can be many reasons why those feelings are present in your life. Your feelings are valid. Feelings are not wrong. But feelings can become a problem when they rule your life.

You can decide to show up even when your emotions tell you to just stay on the sidelines. You can decide to live a life of balance even though you might not feel like it.

When Feelings Follow Faith

The Bible gives us an example of what showing up looks like. The people of Israel were on the road to a much better place, but a huge obstacle lay in their path. They had a decision to make. They could let their feelings get the better of them and run away, or they could act on truth regardless of their feelings.

The Jordan River lay ahead of them. But it was the Jordan River during the harvest months—and that meant flood stage. The river surged and foamed as the waters rushed by. Logs and sticks and dirt and mud—all flew down the Jordan in this season. It would be impossible for the Israelites to cross the river on foot. *How will we ever get across?* the Israelites groaned.

And that was only the half of it. Beyond the Jordan River lay the Promised Land that God had given to them. Once they crossed the Jordan, they would be one step closer to living the life they were meant to live. But who knew what they would find? Probably more challenges, more obstacles—*For heaven's sake, weren't there giants in the land?*

Would the Israelites trust God and cross the Jordan? The Israelites had wandered for years. They had spent a lot of time in the wilderness. But always they had this dream—they knew that a better place existed. It was the land flowing with milk and honey, and the Lord had told them that one day that land would be theirs.

To get there, however, they had to cross this huge river.

The Israelites had several choices: They could choose to run away, to believe that God was dead and there was no hope; they could be nervous and scared and hightail it back to the desert; or they could be complacent and careless and sit around by the river bank and do nothing.

God told them that *now* was the time to act. Their real decision was whether or not to act on truth regardless of their feelings and choose the way of deliverance.

What did the Lord specifically command Joshua and the Israelites to do? Joshua 3:8 records God's words: "When you reach the edge of the Jordan's waters, go and stand in the river."

Go and stand in the river? What kind of plan was that?!

Once more, Israel's faith was put to the test. Here's that fundamental question again that we raised in chapter 1—Did they really believe that *God was good*? Would God abandon them? Would He ignore them? Was He tricking them into taking a dangerous pathway? Or was the invitation to get their feet wet an invitation from a good God who loved His people and had a plan and a future for them?

In the journey toward living a balanced life, there will be many times when God asks us to step into the Jordan at flood stage as a sign of our belief that He is good. Everything in front of us may look confusing or scary or muddy or full of destructive, moving debris. But God assures us that even though we don't know how to get through, He does.

What does He want us to do?

He wants us to show up. He wants us to wade into the river and get our feet wet. That's what happened to the Israelites.

Joshua 3:15 records the outcome: "As soon as the priests who carried the ark reached the Jordan and their feet touched the water's edge, the water from upstream stopped flowing. It piled up in a heap a great distance away . . . [and] the people crossed over."

What is the Lord asking you to do today?

God's invitation to you is to step into the water and make the decision that you want to change. To be willing again and again to take whatever steps are necessary to live this new life. You may not do everything right all the time, but even if you get off track, when you do show up, you are showing your determination to learn how to get back on track and stay on track until your life is changed for the better.

Let's put this principle to the real-life test. In the spaces below, take stock of your life. Write down some thoughts that will help you apply this biblical truth.

Right now, I believe that God is calling me to a new (or renewed) place of health. God's call to me is to step into the Jordan, to get my feet wet, to show up. I may not feel like showing up all the time, but that's okay. Living life emotionally balanced means that I can choose to act in a positive way no matter how I feel.

I know that the Lord is inviting me to . . .

_____

_____

_____

Not showing up looks like . . .

_____

_____

Showing up means that I will . . .

_____

_____

The Healthy Emotional Choice

Let's talk about one very specific place of health to which you're invited to come right now. At First Place 4 Health, each session is 12 weeks long. We ask people to attend one meeting per week. Being accountable by showing up and interacting with others who are following the same path allows you to take your first steps toward living a life with healthy emotional balance.

You may not always feel like going to the meeting, but my encouragement to you is to choose to make that meeting a regular part of your life. There will always be some sort of nagging voice that tells you to stay home. *The meeting's too far. I've been in the car all day. I haven't lost any weight. I want to watch TV tonight.* Regardless of how you're feeling—come. Just come. Don't let emotions rule your life. Rather, act on the knowledge that this meeting is one important factor in your journey. Plan to show up every week.

What will happen at the meeting?

The meeting will last for 1 hour and 15 minutes.

- During the first 15 minutes, a First Place 4 Health leader will weigh you to check your progress each week. You'll be invited to say a memory verse you learned during the week and to hand in your Live It Tracker—an accountability tool that helps you record your progress in achieving balance with your food choices and daily physical activity. Then your leader will return your Live It Tracker from the previous week. This isn't a time of judgment. You're not being graded or reprimanded. The Live It Tracker is a tool to help you on your journey.

- During the next 15 minutes, you'll receive specific training on various health principles, such as eating right and exercising.

- The middle 30 minutes is spent in a Bible study. A First Place 4 Health leader walks the group through the week of study you've just finished, asking questions to help you apply to your life what you've learned. The Bible study time is when you have the opportunity to share what God is teaching you. The last 15 minutes is spent in a prayer time when members can talk about their needs and ask other group members to pray for them.

That's it.

When you attend a weekly First Place 4 Health meeting, you will meet people who are wrestling with the same issues that you are. This meeting is not the same as a church service. At church, you can hear a good message, but you can still attend anonymously, Sunday after Sunday. If someone passes you in the hallway at church and asks how you're doing, it's easy to give a quick "Fine" in passing and never give it a second thought.

At a First Place 4 Health weekly meeting, everyone has openly admitted to having a problem with weight control—and to struggling with living a balanced life. All are journeying this road together. These weekly groups reflect the beauty of the Body of Christ. The people in a First Place 4 Health group cheer you (and you them) to success.

That's what the groups are all about.

Why are these groups so important?

Maybe you think of yourself as the lone wolf when it comes to living healthy; but frankly, I haven't known many people who can achieve balance by themselves. It's difficult to get started. It's difficult to hold yourself accountable. It's easy to feel discouraged and quit at the first sign of difficulty.

We all need other people as we walk toward a healthy lifestyle. Think of your fellow group members—and the weekly First Place 4 Health meeting—as a ready-made accountability system for you. Accountability is so essential in this process of achieving balance. It simply means that you invite someone to walk the road with you.

Speaking for myself, I know that I can't walk this road alone, so I have accountability built into almost every area of my life. I *want* accountability, because it helps bring balance to my life.

When I cross the Jordan, I know I'm not crossing it alone.

Show Up Today

Will you do it? Will you show up?

Showing up is a must for achieving emotional balance. If you show up, you take control of your feelings—you consciously choose to do what is good for you. And that's part of living a balanced life.

Whatever "raging river" is in front of you today, God's invitation to you is to wade into it. Just show up and watch a good God at work in your life.

Checklist for Success

- If you find yourself unwilling to even begin this journey, tell our loving God, and give Him permission to make you willing to be willing.

- Showing up is a key decision that will help you achieve emotional balance. You show up when you're willing to do the hard work needed to achieve a lifestyle change.

- Showing up isn't a one-time act. You are invited to continually make choices that are good for you—to show up once a week for 12 weeks.

- Whenever you show up, you take control of your feelings. You may not *feel* like showing up, but you have the choice to do so anyway. You have the power to consciously choose to do what's good for you. That's an important part of living a balanced life.

• Your specific invitation is to show up weekly at a First Place 4 Health meeting. There you will find the support, encouragement and accountability you need to travel this journey.

Chapter 4

The S.S. Encouragement

Imagine two huge ocean-going vessels.

The first is a luxury liner. Destination: Good Times. It could be sailing to a tropical port or around the world; it could be cruising to Alaska or the Bahamas. It doesn't really matter.

The passengers who board this vessel are given only one instruction. Everything they do on this ship, every activity, every attitude, every thought, every action, everything they say and do and feel must be inspired by this one directive: This cruise is all about *you*.

So the passengers respond accordingly. On the first day they sleep in late then amble to the breakfast buffet where they gorge themselves. Then they stroll to the pool, slather on suntan oil and promptly fall asleep. They awaken famished for a snack, so they clap their hands for a waiter to bring them drinks and pastries. Lunch is another huge buffet. More naps and snacks until dinner—a sumptuous all-you-can-eat feast. Then the lights go down for a fabulous high-class entertainment show in the theater, leaving the passengers calling for more. There's a dessert buffet after the show. Then it's bedtime. If the passengers wake up in the wee hours, there are several all-night diners open with the food piled high. At any time on the cruise, if the music isn't right, an attendant will change it. If a sunshade needs adjusting, a staff member will take care of it. If a pillow needs fluffing, someone else will do that.

This pattern goes on day after day after day.

At the end of the voyage, the passengers have developed a cruise-ship mindset. They are used to eating as much as they want whenever they want. Their definition of "normal" is eating all day, lying around and being entertained. They have developed a 24-hour attitude of "It's all about me"—they expect to be catered to. If something isn't up to snuff, the passengers voice their complaints.

Why? That's what they're supposed to do. This ship has only one rule: *It's all about you.*

Contrast that scenario with what takes place on the second ship, a military carrier. This particular vessel is heading out on an assignment to bring food, medical supplies, protection and encouragement to people in need. This ship has the full support of its government and democratic populace.

On this ship, crew members are given only one instruction. Every activity, every attitude, every thought, every action, everything they say and do and feel must be inspired by this one directive: *This voyage is all about The Mission.*

The crew members respond accordingly. Their sleep pattern is prudent; they eat meals that fuel them for their tasks; they participate as individuals and as a team on assignments that help fulfill their calling. No one caters to them—they take the responsibility to do things for themselves and for the good of the assignment. Sure, they participate in leisure activities, but even their leisure has a purpose—to refresh their minds and bodies so that they can return to their tasks with a new sense of purpose and energy.

At the end of this voyage, the crew members look back on a job well done. They take pride in knowing they have lived with initiative, health and vigor. They feel a sense of accomplishment and purpose. They choose not to evaluate the voyage based on their preferences (whether or not they liked something); rather they base their evaluation on the goals of their mission (did they accomplish what they set out to do?).

Here's my point: Some of you are living life as if you're on a cruise ship. You complain and feel bloated, listless and purposeless. The voyage you've chosen is only making you miserable.

I see this attitude in a lot of different places: employers frustrated by employees; church congregations divided; families unhealthy and depressed; marriages hurting and fractured; individuals aimless and filled with despair—all because of a cruise-ship mindset and the accompanying "all about me" habits.

There is no gentle way to say this. If a cruise-ship outlook characterizes your life, then it's time for the cruise to end—it's time to change ships. There's another ship sailing, and this one is on a mission. It's a military carrier, and the battle is for your health.

This other ship's calling is part of the plan to help you live a balanced life of purpose and wholeness—the life that you truly want, the life you were designed to live.

This new ship is sailing right now. Climb aboard!

When a Mission Is Needed

Boarding the new ship involves your willingness to disembark the one you've been on. You can do that when you truly see and understand the destructive nature of the cruise-ship mindset.

One of the biggest problems with a cruise-ship mentality is that it wreaks havoc on your emotions. A cruise-ship mentality caters only to your feelings. It asks only one question: What do you *feel* like doing? You'll filter everything through your expectation that you deserve to be catered to. And you'll evaluate the world through a mindset that asks: *Did I like how this made me feel?*

As you read in the last chapter, the body wants to do what the body wants to do. With a cruise-ship mentality, your body will seize that one desire of letting feelings rule and run with it to your destruction.

Why eat a healthy salad if there's a stack of doughnuts around? Why get up and read your Bible when you could spend an extra 15 minutes in bed? Why attend a weekly First Place 4 Health meeting when you could relax and watch TV for a couple of hours?

If you let your feelings rule, they will typically choose immediate gratification. But that mindset will only make you feel miserable in the end.

To approach life by letting your feelings rule is one of the most destructive things you can do. Feelings are not wrong, but they always need to be guided by the wisdom and truth found in Scripture. The Bible sets out guidelines with instructions, invitations and warnings so that we can know how to truly live.

In the last chapter, you read that one of the primary ways to bring balance to your emotions is *to show up*, a metaphor used for your willingness to get up and begin again every time you are tempted to quit.

You need to be willing to consciously decide to walk the journey toward living a balanced life. You make that decision more than once. In fact, you will make that decision again and again.

A problem emerges when people think of showing up as the same thing as boarding a cruise ship. This happens sometimes when people first begin First Place 4 Health. And I'll admit that I had this mentality when I first joined the program. My mindset was still dominated by the belief "This is all about me." I boarded the First Place 4 Health program with a cruise-ship mentality.

My reason for joining First Place was anything but spiritual. I had run into a friend at a baby shower. Kay and I had grown up together at Houston's First Baptist Church, but we had not seen each other in quite a while. When I saw that she had lost weight and looked wonderful, I exclaimed, "How could you lose weight and not tell me?!" Kay smiled and said, "Carole, we're going to be 40 next year. Do you want to be fat and 40?" Well, that statement had a ring to it that I didn't like; so when I saw the advertisement for First Place, I decided that it might be the way I could lose weight before I turned 40.

I knew nothing about balanced living. My whole life had been characterized by spurts of grandeur. I had been on a million diets before. One diet called for eating a different food every day. All I remember about that one is that one day I ate nothing but bananas—I don't remember if I lost weight on it or not. If I did, I undoubtedly gained it back. I had been losing and gaining the same 20 pounds for years.

This time, one of my first goals for losing weight was to run a mile—as quickly as I could. I hadn't run in years, but as soon as I set the goal for myself, I jumped in my car and measured off a mile, then came back and laced up my shoes and hit the pavement. A mile was three times around our block. I ran at night so that no one would see me. I wheezed and gasped and huffed and puffed. I set each streetlight as a goal—if I could just make it to that next streetlight . . .

Well, after a few weeks, I finished the mile . . . and never ran again.

On the outside, I had all my spiritual ducks in a row. I taught Sunday School. I was always nice to people (I thought) and hospitable. But my spiritual life was completely out of balance. Very seldom did I actually read my Bible. My prayer life was almost zero. I had a long list of things I had told God I'd absolutely never do. I was positive that if I gave God an inch, He'd send me to the jungles as a missionary. There was no way I was going to do that!

As I continued in the First Place program, God used a series of events to show me that His hand is gentle in our life. He doesn't force change on us. He didn't want to send me to Africa. He wanted to mold me into the woman He designed me to be.

Over time, and through the power of Scripture and the help of my friend Dotty Brewer, I came to see that my cruise-ship mentality would never bring about the lasting change I so desired. I needed to disembark my cruise ship and climb aboard the vessel that invited me on an amazing mission. The mission wasn't about getting my needs met; it was about being who God wanted me to be—someone who loved Him wholeheartedly and loved others as I loved myself (see Matt. 22:37-39).

That's the core teaching of First Place—in fact, this scriptural outlook is where First Place 4 Health derived its name. The First Place part means that you give Christ *first place* in your life. None of us is on the throne of our life; God is! Loving the God of the universe becomes our number-one goal. Loving others created in God's image becomes the outworking of that goal.

Matthew 6:33 is where we find this specific invitation to put Christ first:

> But seek first His kingdom and His righteousness, and all these things will be given to you as well.

That's the call—seeking Christ and His kingdom first. It is only when Christ holds *first place* in your life that everything else has an opportunity to shift toward balance.

So what does changing ships look like? How can you board the ship with a mission? How can you leave behind the attitude that life is all about you?

The answer lies in one simple word: *encouragement.*

Aboard the S.S. Encouragement

Encouragement is defined as adopting the attitude of loving God and loving others, and basing everything we do and say on this foundation.

Health begins when you *show up*; but you can show up at First Place 4 Health with an attitude that shouts "What's in it for me?" That attitude will never bring about the lasting change you desire.

Your invitation in Hebrews 10:25 is twofold: Scripture invites you first to show up—*do not give up meeting together.* The specific context in this verse applies to the temptation in the Early Church for believers to disband and go back to their old beliefs. The application of this verse for us extends to the temptation we might have to quit, to give up, to stop showing up; it invites us to pursue a continued determination to live the way God invites us to live—with health, purpose and direction.

Second, this Scripture invites you to *encourage one another*. We are to love God and love others. Adopting a mindset of encouragement is part of any successful journey toward health. Encouraging someone gives you a task, a purpose—something to do beyond yourself. When you reach beyond yourself, that action circles back to help you as well.

People are lonely and discouraged today. They need to hear and feel your encouragement as much as you need theirs. When people show up to a place of goodness or health with the goal of encouraging one another, the results can be electric—a blessing both given and received. You see, loving God and loving others is in your best interest. This is the way you were meant to live. That's why it's so satisfying to do.

I see examples of this all the time in our First Place 4 Health weekly meetings. A woman who came to my group heard another woman talk about how hard it was to exercise. For physical reasons, walking wasn't an option. The woman offered to be her exercise partner, and the two joined a YMCA to do water aerobics together three times a week.

What if you show up and encourage someone else, but nobody encourages you? That's the cruise-ship mentality. Your path to health starts by loving God and loving others. Your mission is to keep coming and to keep encouraging. Remember, someone needs you. You find purpose and meaning when you encourage others—and purpose and meaning is a reward by itself.

Encouragement is never about a perfectly reciprocal exchange, nor is it meant to be. But after a while, things even out. Whenever you adopt the mindset of encouraging others, encouragement filters back to you somewhere down the line.

Encouragement can take the form of the simplest things—an affirming word, a compliment graciously given, an act of kindness. Or encouragement can become something larger and help us through our toughest times.

A woman in my group had shoulder surgery and was unable to drive. Two other group members took turns taking her to physical therapy every week until she was better. It was a small act of kindness, but they said it helped them see Christ more.

Several years ago, a First Place leader's adult daughter died in a tragic car accident. The daughter and her husband were delivering Christmas presents when their van was hit and both were killed. During the seasons of grieving that followed the loss of her only child, the mother said her First Place 4 Health family was a lifeline. Group members called, wrote cards of encouragement and brought her meals. Now she is a tremendous encouragement to others in times of grief. She can understand because she's been there. Encouragement always circles back.

When we start to love each other as Christ loves us, that's when encouragement can really begin to bloom.

The Smallest Steps

Maybe the idea of being an encouragement to other people is new to you. You wonder how to go about it, even where to start. We are offered some practical guidelines in 1 John 3:16-18.

The first way to become an encourager is to continue to fall in love with Christ. As you learn more about the character and ministry of Jesus Christ, you can't help but follow His lead.

This is how we know what love is: Jesus Christ laid down his life for us. And we ought to lay down our lives for our brothers (1 John 3:16).

The phrase "lay down your life" can sound ominous, but really it's the hallmark of emotional health. In contrast, when your life is ruled by your feelings, you'll do everything else except lay down your life; your primary goal is to gratify your feelings. When you follow the call of Christ to consider the needs of others, you continually ask yourself, *What is the most loving thing I can do for this person?* And then you act on it.

Laying down your life for someone doesn't mean that you fix the person or solve the person's problems or feel the person's pain as if it were your own. But it does mean that you continually act toward others within the bounds of love.

The next verse gives an example of what that might look like. First John 3:17 says:

If anyone has material possessions and sees his brother in need but has no pity on him, how can the love of God be in him?

This is where encouragement becomes very tangible. Is someone in need? Help the person in whatever capacity you can. Material possessions can include any goods or services that money can buy: food, clothes, transportation, shelter, medical care, haircuts, time. If someone you know is lacking in these things, you have the power to encourage that person.

Encouragement is something more than material—it's also spiritual. When we pray for the needs of others, whether during our private prayer time or in a First Place 4 Health group setting, we invite the Lord to be present in the life of those for whom we are praying. Telling someone "I prayed for you today" is often the greatest encouragement we can give.

The last verse—1 John 3:18—offers a self-check of encouragement:

Dear children, let us not love with words or tongue but with actions and in truth.

In other words, don't just talk about encouraging someone; do it. Certainly, encouragement can come in the form of a note, a card or an email. But this verse invites you to go further and to touch the lives of others through bold, loving action.

In her book *Confessions of a Good Christian Girl*, speaker and television personality Tammy Maltby[1] talks about a time when the Lord invited her to encourage someone she didn't know. The encouragement Tammy offered didn't seem like a big deal to her at the time. It was just one small step she had taken to make someone else's life a bit easier.

One afternoon, Tammy was in the checkout line at the grocery store when her attention gradually focused on the woman in front of her. At first glance, it was a woman with whom Tammy thought she had nothing in common. The woman sported piercings in various parts of her body. Her hair was dyed several different colors. Tattoos adorned her arms, legs and neck.

The only thing Tammy could relate to was that the woman had a baby with her, and the child was obviously having a bad day. The baby was screaming. The young mother looked exhausted. She kept sorting through food stamps and figuring out what she could afford and what she had to put back.

Tammy looked at the young mother with the eyes of the Holy Spirit and saw a heart in need of encouragement. So Tammy spoke to her—a little nervously at first. She asked the woman about her baby and volunteered to hold the child as the mother finished going through the checkout line.

Nothing much happened after that. The two women chatted as the line progressed. Tammy told the young mother that her baby was adorable. The young mother collected her child and left. Tammy finished checking out and walked to her car.

Out of nowhere, the young mother appeared again. She ran up to Tammy and said, "I just have to thank you. That's the most encouragement I think I've ever had in my whole life."

Her whole life? Tammy's heart nearly broke to realize how difficult life must be for the young woman. But she also had to smile at the joy of being God's point person—of being the embodiment of His loving encouragement to that young mom.

Tammy hugged the young mother and whispered a few more words of encouragement. One small step—speaking to someone in line at the grocery store—had done so much more than Tammy could imagine. The experience was an incredible encouragement to Tammy, too.

Acting in word and deed is the true meaning of encouragement.

Your Plan Today

Let's put this principle into action. In the spaces below, take stock of your life. Write down some thoughts that will help you apply this principle today.

I believe the Lord is calling me to show up with an outlook of encouragement at . . .

_____

_____

_____

_____

One way I can do this is by . . .

_____

_____

_____

_____

How do you begin to achieve emotional balance in your life?

You begin by choosing to not let your feelings rule your life. You make a decision to head in a healthy direction. And not only that, but you also choose to show up without a cruise-ship mentality. You choose to show up with a selfless attitude—one that seeks to encourage others.

If you show up and encourage someone, you will receive the benefits as well. So come aboard and expect great things to happen.

Checklist for Success

· Showing up is key to achieving emotional balance. You show up when you are willing to do the work it takes to make a lifestyle change.

· When you choose to show up, you need to ditch the cruise-ship mentality and think instead of the mission mindset.

· When you show up focused on encouraging others, you are being faithful to your mission, which is to find emotional health.

· It doesn't take much to encourage others, but whatever you do, be prepared to back up your words with actions.

Note
1. Tammy Maltby with Anne Christian Buchanan, *Confessions of a Good Christian Girl* (Nashville, TN: Thomas Nelson, 2007), n.p. Story used by permission of the author.

First Place 4 Health in Real Life

Becky Turner
Houston, Texas

It was another January, and the scales read over 200 pounds once again. I looked to the heavens and cried out, "God, is this the only thing You can't deliver me from? Is gluttony the 'thorn in the flesh' I will have to deal with all of my life?"

In His gracious and benevolent way, God quickly corrected me on a few things: (1) There is nothing from which He can't deliver me; (2) He desires my cooperation in this process. He wants me to push away from the table sooner, make wiser food choices and begin exercising; (3) Food had become my idol and replaced Him.

I had just moved to a new city, and I was lonely. A typical evening for me was to swing past the Mediterranean buffet place and overeat, then go home, call my friends and whine about how miserable I was. I ran to food for comfort, security and entertainment. I knew that God wanted me to be healthier, that I needed to honor God with my body, because my body is the temple of the Holy Spirit.

So, after much confessing and repenting, I started on a 1,400-calorie-per-day diet, enlisted a personal trainer and began working out seven to eight times a week. Over the next five months, I lost 15 pounds, but then I plateaued. I was still tracking at 1,400 calories and working out, but the weight wasn't coming off.

That summer, the director of the First Place 4 Health ministry at my church asked if I would be a leader the next semester. This was not a total surprise, because I had served in this role many years back.

Although eating 1,400 calories was not a problem for me, the problem was BREAD—my personal drug of choice. Since abstinence is easier for me than balance, I simply had eaten no carbs, or very few carbs, for months. But as I familiarized myself once again with the Live It food plan, I knew that I would need to incorporate breads into my meals so that I could have a balanced diet. To my surprise and joy, the pounds began to drop off. I not only added the bread back into my diet, but I also started to really focus on Scripture memory. By the middle of that fall, I had lost another 20 pounds, memorized 80 Scripture verses and gained lifelong friends!

The weight loss provided me with opportunities to speak about the grace of God. People would ask, "How did it happen? How did you do it?" My standard answer became, "God delivered me." Food was no longer my best friend, my god, or the teddy bear I ran to when I needed comfort. By the power of the Holy Spirit, I was given the ability to say no to ungodliness—which for me had included gluttonous eating, unhealthy foods, eating when not hungry. I was finally free—but it's still a daily process.

For most of us, the difficulty is not losing the weight, but maintaining it. True deliverance for me came not when I reached the goal but when I maintained my goal. This is where lifelong friends became critical for me. I am so grateful that the Bible tells us that "iron sharpens iron" (Prov. 27:17) and that "the blows of friends are better than the kisses of enemies" (see Prov. 27:6, paraphrased). To help me live out this lifestyle of deliverance, God provided three friendships that at times caused sparks to fly, but I knew these people were true friends and they only had my best interests at heart.

First, there was a wiser, older woman who had lived this lifestyle of health for many years. We began to meet as often as possible—usually each weekday—to exercise, quote Scripture verses and pray. We saw many speedy answers to prayer, and I believe that our sacrifice of exercise may have moved the hand of God to act more quickly than He otherwise would have.

Another godly friend helped me remember who I was not. I was no longer a fuzzy, ground-crawling caterpillar. I was transformed into a beautiful monarch butterfly! She did this in many different ways, but one of the greatest ways was by helping me shop and pick out clothes.

Because I am strong-willed and stubborn, I needed a third encourager. Specifically, I needed a "Nathan" in my life, like the prophet Nathan was to King David. A "Nathan" is a person who points out sin and weakness but then walks alongside to help you make it right. Even

Before	After

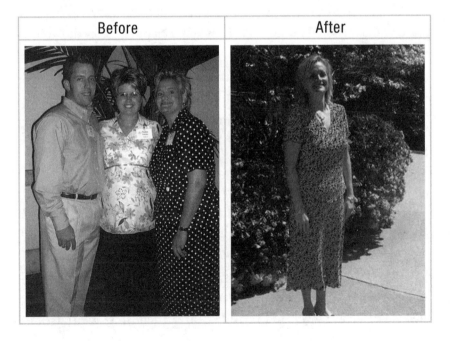

though my Nathan lives hundreds of miles from me, she's the one to whom I fax my Live It Tracker. She's the one who contacts me and asks me if I've exercised that day.

In my pride, I wish I could do it all on my own, but it really does take a community. I thank God for the First Place 4 Health community. It makes deliverance, freedom and abundant living not just a theological concept but also a day-in, day-out reality. I am still a work in progress, but I'm not where I used to be. And through God's grace and the gift of accountability, I will never go back to that place again.

Abby Meloy
Lake City, Florida

Almost eight years ago now, God brought First Place 4 Health into my life, and I am forever grateful. I was a very skeptical, overweight pastor's wife. I had tried many different weight-loss programs, including Christian ones, but I continued to fail; that is, until I had the chance to join First Place.

It all began when some women in my church approached me to ask about starting a First Place 4 Health program here at New Life Church in Lake City. I suspected that this program would involve measuring food portions and complicated numbers, and I'm not fond of dealing with numbers, especially when it comes to food. Obligation got the better of me in the end. I was the pastor's wife; I was overweight; and the women of the church were begging for this program, which they assured me was amazing. So I said we would *try it.*

I felt like I had already tried everything, so why would this program work? Well, 13 weeks later, and 27 pounds lighter, I was completely proven wrong. In this experience of lightening up, I gained a new perspective of what God could do in the realm of my body if I would just trust Him, adding His Word to a balanced way of eating.

Before	After

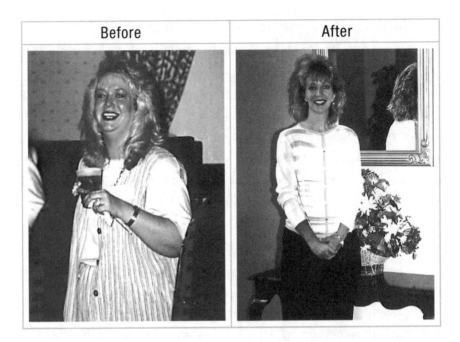

I'm not saying I'm never tempted anymore, because trust me, I'm tempted just like everyone else; though now I know how to handle the temptations. Just going back to reread Carole Lewis's book *Back on Track*, along with the support of all my First Place 4 Health pals, makes staying on track easy.

I have lost 70 pounds through the First Place 4 Health program, and I thank God for all I've been taught spiritually, as well.

Beth Ivey
Columbia, Maryland

I gave my life to Jesus when I was 13, at a Billy Graham Crusade. Although my heart was in it, I don't think I completely got it; so I continued to live the way I wanted to throughout high school and college. After I met the young man who would become my husband, we began attending church together, where I felt Jesus' presence. When I was in church, I really believed, but I would leave Jesus at church.

After my husband and I married, we struggled for six years with infertility, which was the first time in my life that I felt completely helpless. I submitted to God and handed the situation over to Him. He blessed us with two beautiful children.

By this time, I had gained a lot of weight and was again feeling very helpless and negative about myself. Someone had given me a Bible-based weight-loss book, and I thought this was the answer. I called my church with the intention of starting a small group based on this book. The church staff informed me that there was already a weight-loss group that met at my church. Although I wanted to do my own thing, I again submitted to God and joined the existing Bible study.

The day I joined that First Place Bible study was the day that God began to change my life forever. The study was based on Matthew 6:33, which says, "But seek first His kingdom and His righteousness and all these things will be given to you as well." God has completely fulfilled that promise to me. While I have maintained a 35-pound weight loss, He has shown me such joy and peace that the weight loss has become completely secondary to the other changes He has made in my life. He has shown me how to live my life on a daily basis based on His Word; and if I gauge everything I do by that, amazing things happen in my life.

I have been a First Place 4 Health member for more than three years and am the healthiest I have ever been. More important, I am spiritually the healthiest I have ever been. In the summer of 2006, God was speaking to me to start my own First Place 4 Health group. As frightening as that was to me, I was obedient and did just that.

I've been leading my small group of women since then, and as the Lord always does when we are obedient, He has blessed me more than I could have ever imagined. It has been wonderful to see the members grow in Christ and grow closer as a group while gaining success by becoming healthier.

On December 3, 2006, what felt like a pulled muscle in my back developed into a full-blown case of sciatica. For a while I was afraid this injury would be the perfect excuse to go off the program and let Satan sabotage all the hard work I had done. But God has been so merciful, and I know that the First Place 4 Health program is what has prepared me for this experience.

I had been running 3 miles a day, four to five days a week. Now, being so sedentary, I have come up with an "on the floor" exercise routine of movement and stretching that I try to complete daily. I continue to lead the group every week, from the floor! Some of the women brought pillows one week and joined me on the floor!

I am confident that without the relationship I have with Jesus and the First Place 4 Health program, I would be depressed and would eat to excess to deal with my emotions.

God is so good—all the time!

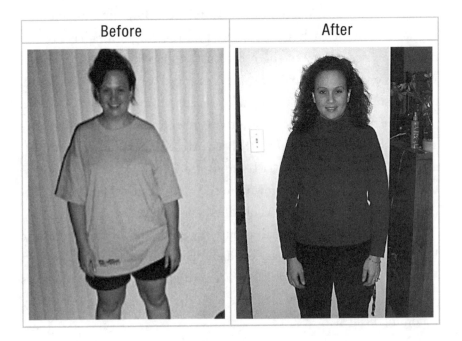

| Before | After |

Bev Henson
Meridian, Mississippi

Have you ever tried to set up a line of dominoes? It can be easy to accidentally hit one while setting them up and have the others fall as well. Or maybe one domino is just a little out of line, and the sequence is unbalanced. My weight-loss "career" has been very much like setting up dominos. I am where I am today with my healthy lifestyle because I have fallen, gotten back up and set myself up again with a deeper knowledge of how to keep the line of my life in order—in balance.

Today I am 54 years old. I have been in an all-out war with my weight since I was 24 years old. My top weight was 310 pounds; my lowest weight on diet pills was 106 pounds (I maintained 106 pounds for about 21 hours!).

For so many years, the "domino" that kept my life from being ordered and balanced was the one that kept telling me I should weigh 106 pounds. The truth was that this was an unobtainable weight goal. Nevertheless, thoughts of that goal became a real stumbling block to me in every diet I tried because I could never reach or maintain it. My thoughts were out of order and so was my heart. I had made up my mind and had set my heart on an unobtainable goal.

At the age of 34, I was radically saved. With His mercy and grace, He began to line up the dominoes in my life that were out of order. I immediately stopped biting my nails and stopped smoking, and God replaced my foul mouth with a mouth full of His words.

However, the one domino that just would not stay in line was my weight. I had the mindset that if my weight was not under control, then nothing in my life was under control. And I didn't think I would have my weight under control until I weighed 106 pounds. I was in serious need of a "heart transplant" to change my heart and a "brain transplant" to renew my mind. Jesus is an awesome transplant surgeon!

In order for my spiritual transplants to be effective, I had to first come to the understanding that the process of transformation is a long one.

For me, joining First Place in July 1997 was the first divine appointment on my journey toward better health. I actually was in First Place for seven months before I got it. I didn't lose a single pound for seven months; on the flip side, I didn't gain any weight. During that seven-month time span, I thought I was spinning my wheels, but actually God was changing my heart and my mind. I was learning, through His mercy and grace, to rest in His arms and stop dwelling on my weight 24/7. I got into His Word through the Bible study and memorizing Scripture, and He began to show me the areas in my life that were so out of order. I hadn't realized there were so many. With the First Place Bible studies, I developed a passion for His words. With the living and breathing Word of God in my life, I began to desire and long for order in my life.

In February 1998, my first mind and heart change occurred. I breathed a sigh of relief when I let go of the goal weight of 106 pounds and set a

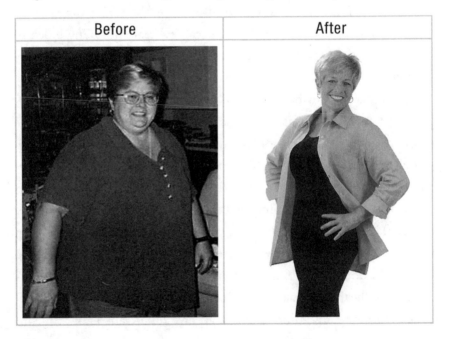

Before	After

new goal of 150 pounds. The next mind and heart change occurred when the Spirit of the Lord took me by the hand, stood me up and told me to start exercising. I stepped out my front door into my promised land on February 8, 1998, and began walking every day.

But soon I longed for more. I always wanted to roller blade or inline skate. I purchased my first inline skates, brought them home and put them on my feet, only to discover that my legs were still so large that I could not fasten the straps. Each Monday I would put my skates on to see if the straps would fasten. A few months later, the straps fastened on my skates. What a feeling of accomplishment! My next moment of change was on a bicycle . . . then a kayak . . . then running, and so on.

God has turned me into a very good senior athlete. I have 15 gold medals and 12 silver medals hanging on a wall over my desk. I compete in mountain biking, kayaking, road biking and power walking. In 2002, I was named Female Athlete of the Year for the state of Mississippi. To God be the glory! Great things He has done!

Here I am, nine years later, and I am still walking in my promised land and possessing it. I haven't fully conquered it yet, but I am far better off than I was that cold February morning in 1998, when I first stepped out my front door. I have failed many times and experienced setbacks and discouragement. But every one of those times when I thought I had messed up, the Holy Spirit was there with a lesson and wisdom to pick me up and move me on.

It is no longer a struggle to stay at my target weight of 150 pounds, and I have come to a place of peace with the scales. I don't beat myself up if my weight is up two or three pounds. Previously, 100 percent of the enjoyment in my life came from food and food events. Today I know that the abundant life is not only about food. It's also about living a healthy lifestyle—and about sharing the beauty of the balanced life with others.

I have been best friends with Zona for 20 years. She is a stay-at-home mom who home schooled all four of her children. When the last child graduated, she took a look at her life and discovered that she had given so much to the children that she had lost some of herself. She was overweight and her life was out of balance. Zona asked me to help her get into shape.

Zona came to my boot camp and began walking. In the beginning, she was very frustrated because she couldn't walk fast or far. She wanted to quit, but I talked to her about pressing on. I told her to stop looking at where everyone else was and concentrate on where she wanted to be. She did press on, and it began to show in every area of her life. She has now lost 40 pounds and looks and feels great. She walks every day and just recently bought a bike.

When her daughter gave birth to a little girl, Zona had to take care of her two-year-old grandson while his mother was in the hospital. Zona called to thank me for helping her get her life in order. She had the energy and endurance to keep up with her grandson for the entire day, and said, "Four years ago I would not have lasted two hours with a two-year-old."

The abundant life that Jesus promised us in John 10:10 is a well-balanced life full of many enjoyable opportunities and enjoyable people. At one time, I had no social life outside of my recliner chair. Today I have so many fun things happening in my life that don't involve food. I now derive great joy from helping others find health and wholeness. The Lord has taken me from sitting to serving.

PART 2

Soul:
Seeking Balance Spiritually

Some people don't believe that being overweight is a spiritual issue. I am acquainted with many men and women who are overweight, and they love and serve God. My personal belief is that being overweight is a fleshly problem with a spiritual solution.

Change begins when you start ingesting truth in your life; and it is God who is the ultimate source of all truth. With Him in your life, every area will begin to come into balance, and the weight issues will be addressed in lasting ways.

What does living a spiritually balanced life look like? That's what we'll discuss over the next three chapters.

Chapter 5

The Pathway of Prayer

When I think of all the things I used to do to try to lose weight . . . ! The one thing I never did at that time was pray about it.

Oh sure, I prayed about other things—asking God to bless the pastor or be with the missionaries overseas. I might have even prayed for a few things for myself, such as my finances (which were an ever-pressing need); my marriage (something I came face to face with every day); my kids (kids always seem to need prayer!).

But pray about my weight? That was something I thought I could handle on my own.

It wasn't that I didn't believe God cared about me; I knew that He did. But my weight was a personal area. I believed that I should practice self-control to lose weight, even though I had lost and gained the same 20 pounds many times. Down deep I figured that God, as ruler of the universe, had a lot of other things more important to deal with than my losing an extra 20 pounds. Weight loss was something I could do by myself. Whatever my rationale, the bottom line when it came to my weight loss was to leave God out of the equation.

How about you? When you take stock of your life, to what degree is God the center and core of all that you do? To what degree do you know—not just in your head but also in your heart—that God loves you and is deeply interested in every facet of your life? To what degree are you comfortable being completely honest with God? Are you willing to be vulnerable in every area of your life as you stand before Him? Do you know that God truly wants the best for you, and can you affirm that with confidence?

I believe that lasting weight loss is dependent on our relationship with God. We can struggle and sweat all we want, and we can count calories and climb stairs, but until we learn to trust Him fully with our life—until we rest in Him and let Him lead us—we will never experience lasting success in this area.

To lose weight, our lives must be in balance spiritually.

The problem is, we seldom think about weight loss in spiritual terms.

The Problem with Surrender

Quick, tell me—if you want to lose weight, what's the first thing you must do?

Did you say "exercise" or "eat less"? Those are what we typically think of when it comes to weight loss. But do you ever think about surrendering your life to Christ as the answer?

It sounds like a strange formula for success—if you want to lose weight, start on your knees—but this is a profound truth I don't want you to miss. The goal in the First Place 4 Health program is not just to lose weight. The goal is to live a balanced life—spiritually, mentally, emotionally and physically. When that happens, the issue of weight loss will be addressed in true, lasting ways. So, when it comes to living a truly balanced life, you can't do it without the Lord.

The idea of surrender does not, at first thought, seem like a positive thing. We're not typically encouraged to surrender to anything or anybody. Surrender is what losing armies do. Surrender is what happens when a child hands over his lunch money to the school bully. Surrender connotes the idea of weakness or loss. When we surrender, it feels like we're losing control—perhaps even losing our identity.

What do we do if we choose not to surrender our life to Christ? Simple—we grab on to our life and squeeze it for all it's worth. We try to live in our own strength. In that scenario, what might your self-talk be? Have you ever said anything to yourself such as

- I don't need God. I can do this on my own.
- My way is best. I don't care what God thinks.
- This is all up to me. No one really cares about me anyway.
- I need to keep my life hidden. No one can know the real me.

Your wording may be different, but it represents the same idea. We have all thought that we can do weight loss without addressing the spiritual aspect of our life. When our life isn't surrendered to God, we mistakenly think that all the power has to come from us.

That just doesn't work.

You've seen the statistics, and they don't look good. The vast majority of weight-loss efforts are doomed. We've tried every quick-fix plan or idea presented in the media. Oh sure, we may lose some weight for a while, but as long as we mistakenly believe that weight loss is all up to us, we will forever regain whatever pounds were shed. Might it be time to consider a better way to tackle the problem?

I invite you to consider the word "surrender" in a whole new light—the light of bringing God into the equation. In fact, God isn't just *one factor* in the equation; He's the sum total of everything on which we stand.

The foundation for surrender to the Lord is found in Matthew 11:28-30, a passage that records Jesus' words:

Come to me, all you who are weary and burdened, and I will give you rest. Take my yoke upon you and learn from me, for I am gentle and humble in heart, and you will find rest for your souls. For my yoke is easy and my burden is light.

When we constantly strive to do something yet do not succeed, we become worn out. We also get weary and burdened when we become tangled in sin, chase after quick fixes or participate in behaviors that bring harm to our life.

In contrast, Jesus offers us true rest. The imagery is of yoking ourselves with Christ—becoming joined with Him and His direction, following His pathways, obeying His commands, learning from His ministry and example. When we follow Christ, we find that His way is restful, even easy and light. Our invitation is to trade our heavy burdens for His way. This is true surrender. And the benefit is all ours.

What does surrender to the Lord look like?

It starts by beginning every day with a simple thought and prayer: *God, this day is for You.* Every day is a new beginning, a new opportunity to dedicate ourselves and our actions to the Lord.

Just start there—*God, this day is for You.* God will show you what to do next.

Calling to God

I thought I didn't need to bother God with my weight loss. God was too busy or too concerned with other things. Besides, I wasn't sure what He might ask me to do if I surrendered every part of my life to Him.

When I began First Place, I believed that God had given me common sense, and He expected me to use it. (By the way, I still believe that.) I knew enough about what His Word says that I knew what to do, but I still acted impulsively many times and made decisions based on my own way of thinking.

God has made tremendous changes in this area of my life. He has taught me to trust Him and His goodness, and to wait on Him for instructions. Following His lead, I've been able to make decisions based on His will, not my own. But I've had to be patient. I've had to be willing to not have answers overnight, because God works in His time, not mine.

I have found great rest in Jeremiah 33:3, in which God says, "Call to me and I will answer you and tell you great and unsearchable things you do not know."

This is God's invitation to us—to always approach God. I look at Jeremiah 33:3 as God's phone number. He's always there, always awake and never too busy to take my call. We can go confidently to the Lord! We can approach His throne of grace with assurance. God loves us. He cares about us. He is deeply interested in every part of our lives, even our issues with weight.

I believe there are areas in which all of us have difficulty surrendering to God. We want to give our lives to Him, but still we hold back. For instance, when I teach my First Place 4 Health class, it's easy to think that everyone's growth depends on me; it's easy to worry and fret about the outcome, to start believing that people will be blessed by what I have to say rather than what is shown to them in God's Word and by the power of the Holy Spirit. Over the years, I've learned to go before God and wait for His guidance in this area. I continue to read and study throughout the week, but I've learned to depend on Him for the final outline. He always comes through. When I trust Him, He always does more than I could ever ask or imagine.

If you are strong-willed like me, God has to show you that His way is best. Eventually you will learn that only by waiting on Him will you receive His best. You need to allow Him to make lasting changes in your life. Those changes probably will not happen overnight. They will happen in His time and in His way.

God will only make those changes when we make good choices. That's part of the paradox—it's all up to God, yet we are still responsible for our decisions. As we make the right choices, God reveals His plan and purposes to us.

I see this happen all the time. When I meet people at First Place 4 Health conferences all over the country, I often ask, "How much weight have you lost?" Many times I hear a testimony such as, "Well, I've lost X pounds. But that's not the most important benefit. I've had a life-changing spiritual experience that's been more valuable to me than weight loss could ever be."

That's what I'm talking about. When your life comes into balance spiritually, the rest falls into place. God shows you how to live in every area of life.

There are three components necessary to spiritual balance. I'd like to touch upon them here and in the next two chapters. The first component is prayer.

Breathing in Prayer

I must admit that when I came to First Place, I had no idea how to pray. I did spontaneous "shoot up" prayers all the time, such as "Lord, I need Your help right now" (which is fine to do), but I seldom spent time truly talking with God. I knew nothing about having deep conversations with the Lord, sitting still with Him, letting Him talk to me. I had not developed a true friendship with God.

First Place 4 Health is all about seeking God before anything else. Each day, the invitation to you and to me is to carve out time to pray. Prayer is such an important part of balance. I find that when I spend time with God daily, He conditions my heart ahead of time to help meet the needs of people I come in contact with. Psalm 32:8 says, "I will instruct you and teach you in the way you should go; I will counsel you and watch over you." What a promise! When we pray, God instructs us, teaches us, counsels us and watches over us.

Jesus is our example of how to live a prayerful life. He spent much time praying alone and in quiet places. One example of this is found in Luke 5:16: "Jesus often withdrew to lonely places and prayed." Obviously, Christ knew the value of not being distracted. We see the evidence of prayer in His life through His close relationship with the Father, His power in accomplishing the Father's will, and His commitment to follow God no matter what the cost.

Prayer gives us access to the Creator of the universe. God loves us so much that He gave us prayer as a way to personally communicate with Him, and He with us. Prayer is God's idea. We pray because we need and want to, but also because God desires communion with us.

Over the years, I have used various means to help me pray. One of the best methods I have found is keeping a prayer journal. I use my journal to write out my prayers to God. Prayer journaling helps me stay focused during my prayer time. Another benefit of keeping a journal is being able to see how God answers prayer—even when you don't realize why you're praying for a certain person or thing.

One morning, I felt led to pray for one of our First Place leaders from another state. When I arrived at work that morning, I sent her a note and told her that I didn't know why she was on my heart that morning, but I had prayed for her. About a week later, I received a note that read, "You will never know what it meant to know that you were praying for me that day." She went on to tell me about the events that were going on in her life and how much turmoil she was in. The Holy Spirit has the power to unite believers through the power of prayer. Our call is to show up for our prayer time each day to allow God to communicate to us regarding the people who need our prayers.

Another way to stay focused is to pray out loud. When Johnny and I moved to Galveston Bay eight years ago, it became harder to write my prayers each morning. I now had a 45-mile commute to work, and I always felt rushed to get on the road. So it was an amazing revelation to me several years ago when Jeannie Blocher, president of Body & Soul Aerobics, and I were in Ventura, California, and we went for a walk, to hear her say, "Why don't we pray about our meetings today as we walk?" She began to pray out loud, and when she would stop, I prayed. When I stopped, Jeannie prayed again. Before we knew it, we had walked and prayed for an hour! I was astounded that I had not discovered this secret of prayer—when you pray out loud, your mind stays focused the same way it does when you write your prayers.

Christ's model of prayer (see Matt. 6:9-13) also teaches you to pray for yourself and ask for your daily bread. Some daily needs are minor and routine, though others may be much bigger.

If you have a close friend, you want to get to know him or her, don't you? You want to tell this person all about your life, and you want this person to do the same. The Lord wants to be your friend. Go to Him, confide in Him. Spend time with Him today.

Getting Personal

Your commitment to prayer is one of the most important steps you'll ever take in the First Place 4 Health program. Your heavenly Father wants a personal relationship with you. He invites you to spend time with Him daily through prayer.

To begin, determine what time of day is best for you to have a quiet time alone with God. Morning is my best time. I wake up alert, so I'm able to give my best to God early in the day. Your life may be different. Perhaps you have small children at home, and no matter how much you try, you cannot get up in the morning before your children. If you identify with this situation, your child's naptime might be when you can have a quiet time with God. Or perhaps you can leave for work early enough to have your quiet time at your desk. If you live alone, maybe you prefer to have your quiet time in the evening. Whenever you meet with God, it needs to be when you can be alone with no (or few) interruptions.

If prayer is new to you, I suggest using the F.I.R.S.T. method of prayer. This is certainly not the only way to pray, but it gives you an easy way to remember some of the important aspects of prayer. Let's take a look at each of these aspects.

F: Focus

It's easier to focus if you have a regular place where you meet with God each day. Find an isolated spot somewhere out of the main traffic area of your home or office so that you will not be interrupted or easily distracted. Keep your Bible, a devotional book, your First Place 4 Health Bible study and prayer journal on a table beside the chair or sofa where you plan to sit. Using the same spot each day will help you focus on why you are there.

For a good devotional book, you might try reading *My Utmost for His Highest* by Oswald Chambers. Use this book to help start your quiet time with God. This classic book never grows stale.

I: Invite

Once you are in your spot, ready to meet with God, the first thing to do is invite Him to join you there. You can do this by singing a praise song or hymn or, if you prefer, write the words of the song or a praise psalm from your Bible in your journal. The purpose of this activity is to take the focus off of you and put it on the greatness of God.

I like to begin my times of prayer with adoration. Adoration simply means to praise. When you begin your time of prayer, start by praising God for His character, for everything He is, and for everything He has done. This might feel awkward to you at first; but with a little practice, you will find that praising God will elevate your mind to the right attitude for prayer.

The Lord's Prayer begins with adoration. Many of us learned this prayer when we were young. It's found in Matthew 6 and Luke 11. It begins, "Our Father, who art in heaven, hallowed be thy name." The word "hallowed" means that something is sacred, honored or blessed. When we say that God's name is hallowed, this is one way of adoring Him.

R: Reconcile

To reconcile is to agree with God that our sin is grievous in His sight. David stated this eloquently in Psalm 32:5: "Then I acknowledged my sin to you and did not cover up my iniquity. I said, 'I will confess my transgressions to the LORD'— and you forgave the guilt of my sin." In the New Testament, the apostle John said the same thing in 1 John 1:9: "If we confess our sins, he is faithful and just and will forgive us our sins and purify us from all unrighteousness."

After asking God to reveal anything you might have done or said in the last 24 hours that wasn't right, and that you need to be aware of, sit quietly before Him. Ask Him to also show you where you neglected to do or say something that was right and would have been helpful to you or to someone else. Paul said it best in Romans 7:15: "I do not understand what I do. For what I want to do, I do not do, but what I hate I do."

After the Holy Spirit reveals any wrong action, attitude of the heart and/or any words or good deeds that you could have said or done but didn't, tell God that you're sorry and ask His forgiveness as well as His help in this area. If your sin involved another person, see if you can arrange a time before you meet with God tomorrow to talk to the person and ask his or her forgiveness too. Reconciling with God and with others keeps us clean and right with God and with other people.

S: Study Scripture

Now you are ready to study Scripture, which is something to be done thoughtfully and prayerfully. You can find out more about studying God's Word in chapter 7.

Jesus said in John 8:32-33, "If you hold to my teaching, you are really my disciples. Then you will know the truth and the truth will set you free."

Studying the Bible teaches you about God and what He desires for your life. Every word of the Bible is true, and this is the reason we study it so that we can replace distorted thinking with the truth.

T: Trust

Finish your time each day by placing your life and daily activities into God's loving hands. Proverbs 3:5-6 are great verses about trust: "Trust in the LORD with all your heart and lean not on your own understanding; in all your ways acknowledge him, and he will make your paths straight."

When we trust God, we acknowledge that we want His schedule to be our schedule today. We say that if He wants to intervene in the plans we have made, it is perfectly all right, because we trust Him to accomplish what He desires for us today.

The F.I.R.S.T. guide for your daily quiet time with God is only a suggestion. It is not the only way to have a quiet time. You are encouraged to make time with God each day a part of your personal lifestyle. Trust that God is interested in spending time with you, and He will help you find the time to spend with Him.

Corporate Prayer

I want to touch on corporate prayer, another part of prayer that you'll encounter at a First Place 4 Health meeting. We believe in the importance of praying together as a group, so we pray at the beginning and at the end of every meeting.

The prayer time at the beginning is usually shorter—often it's simply to commit the meeting to the Lord and ask Him to help us focus on the material at hand.

Usually the prayer time at the end of each meeting lasts about 15 minutes. During this time, participants ask for prayer for themselves or for needs that affect their success in the program. We encourage people to limit prayer requests to personal needs.

As you make yourself vulnerable enough to ask for prayer for your specific needs, you will see the mighty power of prayer at work. For instance, one lady who is in my 6:15 A.M. First Place 4 Health group was having severe marital problems. Sometimes she barely got inside the door before she burst into tears. To attend the meeting, she drove a long way early in the morning. She would literally hold in her tears until she arrived at the meeting and we could surround her and pray with her so that she could face the day. We rallied around this hurting person and encouraged her by praying over her and lifting up her needs to the Lord.

It is important to note here that with corporate prayer we emphasize that prayer requests need to stay inside the group. We ask each participant to never share a prayer request with anyone outside the group. As a result, the members of the group know their requests will remain confidential. From my experience, members honor this request and place the prayer needs in God's capable hands.

When we have a safe place for our requests, we can voice our deep concerns and anxieties—and they cease to have power over us.

Spiritual Balance Today

The core of the First Place 4 Health program is living a life of balance in all areas—the physical, the spiritual, the mental and the emotional. A balanced life is possible only when Jesus Christ is at its center.

God's invitation to you today is to invite Him to be at the center and core of all that you do. The Lord wants you to know—not just in your head but in your heart as well—that His way is best. He wants you to rest assured that He loves you and is deeply interested in every facet of your life.

Take stock of your life today. To what degree are you comfortable with being completely honest with God? Are you willing to be vulnerable in every area of your life as you stand before Him?

His invitation is for you to take His yoke upon you and to learn from Him. His pathway is easy and His load is light. You can begin walking that pathway through prayer.

Checklist for Success

- Change starts when you begin ingesting truth in your life. God is the ultimate source of all truth. With Him, your life will become balanced, and your issues with weight will be addressed in lasting ways.

- When Jesus Christ is Lord of your life, you can approach His throne of grace with assurance. God loves you and cares about you, and He is deeply interested in every part of your life, even your struggle with weight loss.

- Surrender of your life to God begins every day with a simple prayer: *God, this day is for You.* Dedicate every day of your new journey to the Lord.

- If you want to lose weight, start on your knees.

Chapter 6

The Compass of Scripture

The Bible is not a book that is primarily about weight loss. Neither is it a diet book, a cookbook, a medical book or an exercise book. But one of the best ways for you to lose weight is by reading your Bible every day. Remember: You achieve balance by making a series of small positive choices day after day after day. Reading the Bible every day is an important part of living a balanced life.

I like to think of it this way: In the second *Pirates of the Caribbean* movie from Walt Disney Productions, Captain Jack Sparrow carries with him a crazy compass that everyone laughs at because the needle never points north. Viewers soon find out that the compass arrow points in the direction of whatever a person's heart desires. In Captain Jack's case, it's pirate booty. His heart desires the loot.

Many of us are similarly guided. We let our heart's desires dictate what path we will follow. Our desires can be easily shaped by the culture around us, and that culture is not concerned with our best interests.

The culture is not all wrong. It is simply driven by a different set of principles. Mostly, the culture wants to sell us something, and it will make all sorts of false promises to get our money and allegiance.

Where do your desires lead you?

Maybe your compass points you to a well-stocked refrigerator filled with over-salted, over-processed, fat- and sugar-laden foods.

Perhaps your compass points to "the good life," a life filled with too much stuff. Your quest for the good life has resulted in a frenzied work week, not enough sleep and not enough time with your spouse and children, much less time for yourself or for the Lord.

Perhaps your compass directs you to look at exercise and announce, "I could never do that" or "I don't want to do that" or "I'm too old to do that" or "I'll do it later—much later."

Toward what or whom does your compass needle point? Some of the things offered by our culture are not intrinsically wrong, but it's all too easy to let our values, beliefs and desires become shaped by whatever appears alluring. Whenever your compass gets fixed on the wrong goal, the result is an unbalanced life.

That's why Scripture can play such a vital role in helping you live a balanced life. Scripture points your heart to whatever is true, noble and right.

The Bible is the true compass that you and I need to point us in the right direction.

Desires Equal Behavior

Problems emerge whenever a person desires something unhealthy and pursues that desire. What goes into the mind guides our desires, or at least needs to be filtered by our mind; and a long time of filtering junk can wear down the filter. So it makes sense that you need to be very careful with the things you allow into your mind.

The problem emerges like this: You want to lose weight, so your immediate thought is, *How can I shed pounds the quickest way?* You go on some sort of diet and you lose weight for a time, but your mind still desires the unhealthy food you have been eating. Think about it: How many times have you lost weight or finished a diet only to breathe a sigh of relief because now you can go back to eating the way you really want to eat?

You see, most diets only address the outward behavior of what you eat. But a huge part of the equation for weight-loss success includes the question of *why* you eat what you eat. You've got to examine and realign the desires that are guiding your behavior; otherwise you'll return to old habits every time. You've got to get a new compass that points you in the right direction.

Here's how the problem lays out in point form:

- You allow the culture around you to guide your desires.
- You desire what's unhealthy and you form harmful habits.
- The harmful habits create a physical problem: weight gain.
- You address only the weight gain without realigning the desires that drive the habit.
- Sometimes you lose weight for a while, but since your old habits are just under the surface, you return to your habits when the diet is over.

Weight loss will never be lasting unless you examine the desires that guide your unhealthy habits. That's why reading Scripture every day is so important. It realigns your desires and helps you sift through the various messages vying for your attention in our culture.

Are you still thinking that you aren't shaped by your culture? Think again. What's the first thing that comes to mind when I mention the words:

Tide.

Cheer.

All.

Gain.

Go down the line. If you're like me, you didn't think of the ocean's movement or an optimistic feeling or a total amount or an increase. What did you think of? Laundry detergent—plain and simple. Why? Because all around you, every day, you are bombarded with messages about what you should desire. Culture is always switched on. You can't escape it. And though it's not all bad, it does want you to do what it wants you to do.

Let's take a look at a biblical example of how a culture can position itself to shape a person's desires.

In about 586 B.C., Nebuchadnezzar, king of Babylon, came to Jerusalem with a vast army and besieged the city. Jerusalem fell and Nebuchadnezzar carried back to Babylon all the spoils of the city—gold, silver, animals, and the like. He also took one of the most valuable resources any country has—the young people. He stole the next generation! Daniel 1:4 describes the teens he brought back to Babylon as "young men, without any physical defect, handsome, showing aptitude for every kind of learning, well informed, quick to understand, and qualified to serve in the king's palace."

What was going to happen to these young captives?

Brainwashing.

These kidnapped teenagers were taught the language and literature of Babylon, a country and culture that did not follow the Lord. The teens were assigned a diet from the king's table, food far different from what they were used to eating, and certainly not a meal plan that followed the strict regulations for health set down by Moses. The young people were indoctrinated in the ways of Babylon for three years, after which they would enter the king's service.

Do you see what was happening? Nebuchadnezzar had one goal with these Hebrew young people—he wanted to transform them into good Babylonians. He wanted to immerse them in his culture so that they would think, talk, eat, dress, believe and act the way he wanted.

That's what any powerful culture does.

And that's what your culture is trying to do with you. Your culture wants you to think certain thoughts, desire certain things, adopt certain beliefs and act in a certain way. It will push, pull and persuade you to the place where you desire only what it "feeds" you.

The good news in Daniel's case is that he chose to make a stand for truth. He didn't ignore his new culture. He didn't even battle against it. But he kept himself grounded by what he knew was true. He kept praying. He kept his heart devoted to the Lord. Specifically, Daniel proposed a 10-day test that would turn the culture of Babylon on its head.

For 10 days, Daniel and his three Hebrew friends, Hananiah, Mishael, and Azariah, respectfully asked to be taken off the king's heavy diet and placed back on the healthy diet they had always known. Some Bible translations translate this diet as vegetables only, which conjures up images of Daniel eating salad. But the word in the original language is actually "pulse," a broader word that encompasses a variety of sown foods such as grains and legumes. (Some types of meat were permitted in Hebrew culture; but we're not sure if Daniel's diet also included meat when he was in Babylon.) The bottom line is that Daniel asked to eat only in a way that was vital and vibrant, as a healthy heartbeat or "pulse" would be. Scripture records the outcome of the test in Daniel 1:15:

> At the end of the ten days they looked healthier and better nourished than any of the young men who ate the royal food.

God blessed Daniel and his three friends while they lived in Babylon. The teens were given knowledge and understanding. When they were tested before the king, none were found to be equal to them.

This is the way of walking in the truth.

Your call as a believer is not to make a stand *against* your culture. Christ's call to you is higher than that—He wants you to make a stand for truth *within* your culture. Matthew 5:13-14 invites you to be "salt and light"—someone who makes an impact for truth. Being salt and light doesn't mean that you need to hate your culture or run from it; but it does mean that you recognize the culture's pull, and you choose to follow the truth regardless of what that culture tells you.

Christ's invitation is radical. He wants you to know the truth, be set free by the truth and help others to be set free by the truth. There's only one way to do that. To know what truth is, you need to read God's Word.

True Spiritual Balance

How does reading Scripture help you lose weight and keep it off?

Spiritual balance happens when your mind and heart are filled with good things, not swayed by the culture. When you know Scripture, you can align your desires with truth. The Bible points your compass in the right direction. Your heart's desires will be for good things, not for things that harm you. When voices from our culture tell you which way you should go, Scripture helps you stand for truth within the midst of those voices. Scripture attacks unhealthy practices and changes them from the inside out so that real change can occur in lasting ways.

Psalm 1:1-3 puts it this way:

Blessed is the man
Who does not walk in the counsel of the wicked
Or stand in the way of sinners
Or sit in the seat of mockers.
But his delight is in the law of the LORD,
And on his law he meditates day and night.
He is like a tree planted by streams of water,
Which yields its fruit in season
And whose leaf does not wither.
Whatever he does prospers.

Godly people are not influenced by an unrighteous culture but by meditating on the Word of God. For all who delight in living by God's Word, there is health and wholeness. The writer of Psalm 1 compares this healthy way of living to a tree planted by the water's edge where it consistently drinks in all the goodness of a flowing stream. That tree bears a good crop and doesn't droop and fade in hard times.

This is the life God calls you to live!

Instead of your heart's desire being for what's in the refrigerator, for instance, perhaps your heart is guided by the compass of Jesus' words recorded in Luke 4:4: "Man does not live on bread alone."

Instead of your heart's desire being captivated by the "good" life (AKA the "frenzied" life), your heart is guided by the compass of Matthew 6:19: "Do not store up for yourselves treasures on earth, where moth and rust destroy, and where thieves break in and steal."

Instead of your heart's desire being guided by a resolution to shun exercise, your heart is guided by Philippians 4:13: "I can do everything through him who gives me strength."

I don't want to oversimplify how Christ might transform your desires, but you get the picture. When you read Scripture, your desires become guided by truth, not culture. And this affects how you live— including how you eat.

Let's think for a moment in some broad-brush strokes about what Scripture is and why it's so necessary for your life.

The Bible Is Divinely Inspired

To begin with, the Bible is divinely inspired. The Bible contains the very words of our everlasting, almighty, all-powerful God. Scripture is not simply wise sayings, inspirational stories or "the good book."

The words of Scripture are the very thoughts of God, as we read in 2 Timothy 3:16-17:

All Scripture is God-breathed and is useful for teaching, rebuking, correcting and training in righteousness, so that the man of God may be thoroughly equipped for every good work.

The phrase "God-breathed" means "inspired." This means that God is the author of Scripture, although He used humans to write it down.

> For prophecy never had its origin in the will of man, but men spoke from God as they were carried along by the Holy Spirit (2 Pet. 1:21).

Note that *all* of Scripture is useful. This means that you can read from anywhere in the Bible and it will benefit you in some way. People often think they need to read from one of the "mainstay" books in the Bible—something meaty like Romans, or complex like Revelation. But the *entire* Bible is useful.

Looking for a love story? Try Song of Solomon.

Looking for action and adventure? Try the book of Joshua.

Looking for a poignant tale of duty, faith and love? Try the book of Ruth.

Everything in Scripture is there for a reason. If you've never explored all the richness in Scripture, I invite you to open up your Bible, walk around in its pages and see the sights. Scripture is full of things you may have never imagined.

The Bible Is Mighty in Its Influence

You can read a stirring book and be motivated to do something important, but the Bible goes beyond that. The Word of God is alive, because with the Word of God comes the influence of the Holy Spirit. I don't think of the Bible necessarily as mystical or magical, but I know that God is alive and that He uses the very pages of Scripture to speak to me and transform my life and heart.

Hebrews 4:12 is the foundational verse that tells us Scripture is more than just a stirring book:

For the word of God is living and active. Sharper than any double-edged sword, it penetrates even to dividing soul and spirit, joints and marrow; it judges the thoughts and attitudes of the heart.

The Bible uses various other word pictures to help describe the Word of God. Jeremiah 5:14 calls it a devouring flame. Jeremiah 23:29 says it is like a hammer. Ezekiel 37:7 describes it as a life-giving force. Romans 1:16 calls it a saving power. Ephesians 6:17 calls Scripture a Spirit-filled sword.

When you are seeking wisdom, consolation and help, the Bible will become a familiar companion that will speak God's words to you in times of trouble. As you read the Bible on a consistent and regular basis, your personal relationship with your heavenly Father will become deeper and more meaningful. Prayer is speaking to God, but Scripture reading is God speaking to us. And His Word is alive!

The Bible Is Food for Your Soul

Just as you must eat food to physically stay alive, you need to eat the Word of God to nourish your inner life. The Bible is food for your soul.

Your natural inclination is to get up each day and approach the world on your own, where pressures inevitably will cloud the day and cause a variety of anxieties. The better way is to start each day by letting Scripture focus your view so that you can see the world through the eyes of Christ. Your invitation is to return to this source of spiritual food again and again.

Deuteronomy 8:3 describes Scripture as life-giving and sustaining. Job 23:12 encourages you to "treasure the words of his mouth more than [your] daily bread." Psalm 119:103 takes the idea further and describes Scripture as "sweeter than honey." Jeremiah 15:16 calls the

Word of God a joy and a delight. First Peter 2:2 describes Scripture as "pure spiritual milk," the absolute essential nutrients every human needs to survive.

The Bible Is a Light for Your Path

The Bible is a book of wisdom and direction, filled with practical advice and examples of how people lived out their faith. Scripture illuminates the rocky terrain and the darkened alleyways of your life. It keeps you from evil and guides your journey.

Psalm 19:8 says:

The precepts of the LORD are right,
giving joy to the heart.
The commands of the LORD are radiant,
giving light to the eyes.

Much of the book of Proverbs describes how biblical wisdom can keep a person from danger and destruction. Proverbs 6:23 says:

For these commands are a lamp,
this teaching is a light.

Next Steps

Begin reading God's Word on a daily basis and ask God to give you a love for His Word.

If you are unfamiliar with the Bible, you might begin by reading the Gospel of John. Read this Gospel several times until you understand what it says; then continue with another book of the Bible. Another good and practical place to start reading is in the book of Proverbs.

There is no right or wrong way to read God's Word. The key thing is simply to begin.

I am very grateful for Christian parents who took me to church and taught me to read and study God's Word for direction in life. Your story may be different, and that's okay. You might not own a Bible, or you might have to dust off an old one and take it to the First Place 4 Health group meeting. That's fine. Just start reading your Bible today.

The First Place 4 Health Member's Guide includes a systematic Bible reading plan that will enable you to read the entire Bible in a one-year period. Just look up the particular reading for each day, and do the same the next day and the next.

You can also use a one-year Bible, which is available in any Christian bookstore and offered in several different Bible translations. In a one-year Bible, the Scripture passages are divided each day into a selection from the Old Testament, the New Testament and the books of Psalms and Proverbs. I often use a one-year Bible because I tend to read more using this system.

Your invitation to read Scripture doesn't depend on how much or how little you read each day. Although quantity is not the main issue, I do suggest that you read one to two chapters per day. Reading God's Word will increase your desire to know Him in a deeper way.

As you read, ask God to give you insight from His words to help you in the activities of your day. Sometimes the Holy Spirit might impress you to stop on a particular verse. After you read that verse a few times, God may give you insight into a current problem you're experiencing. He can actually speak to you through a particular verse or passage from His Word.

When I came to First Place, I owned several Bibles; I even carried one to church. I was familiar with Bible stories. But I had never really read the Bible consistently.

Through the influence of the First Place program, the Bible has become my handbook for life. I always begin each day by opening my Bible. It helps to read systematically rather than just reading wherever I land. So I usually read through a book of the Bible before moving on to another one. Before I begin reading, I ask the Lord to show me one verse that I'll specifically need for the day. And He does! Sometimes the verse that is impressed upon my heart is something I will need in a subtle way. Sometimes it's a verse that I meditate on (think about and chew on) throughout the day. Sometimes it's a verse that is carried with me forever.

I've discussed the following story in detail in my book *A Thankful Heart*, but it's such a huge part of my life and illustrates this point so well of taking in God's Word that I just want to mention it here. On Thanksgiving morning 2001, I woke up early, at 4:00 A.M., but felt the temptation to stay in bed. It was Thanksgiving Day, for heaven's sake! But I felt a strong urge from the Lord to get up and read.

I opened my Bible to James 1:2-4: "Consider it pure joy, my brothers, whenever you face trials of many kinds, because you know that the testing of your faith develops perseverance. Perseverance must finish its work so that you may be mature and complete, not lacking anything."

I read those verses, ingested them and stuck them away in the back of my mind, not knowing how much I would need those verses that day. You see, that was the horror-filled day when our daughter Shari was struck by a drunk driver and killed. I stayed in James chapter 1 for three or four months afterward. Somehow, the Lord was telling me that even this was part of His plan. I'm forever grateful that I got up that Thanksgiving morning to spend time in His Word. Several months after Shari died, I realized that the Lord Jesus woke me up early that Thanksgiving morning because He knew what was going to happen that day, and He was grieving what we were going to experience that night and wanted to spend time with me to prepare my heart.

God knows all about your cares and concerns. You have the choice to read His Word. So choose to read His Word every day. His Word is one of the ways He speaks to you. Your invitation is to immerse yourself regularly in His plan for your life as revealed in the Bible.

Your Plan Today

Reading Scripture every day can play a vital role in your living a balanced life. Scripture will point your heart to whatever is true, noble and right, because the Bible is your only true compass. It's the tool you need to live the life you really want to live.

When Scripture is at work in your life, your desires and habits can become cleansed, healed and transformed to the will of God. And one of the results will be lasting weight loss.

Will you begin reading your Bible today?

Checklist for Success

- Being overweight is a fleshly problem with a spiritual solution. Change begins when you start ingesting truth into your life; and it is God who is the ultimate source of all truth. With Him, your life will become balanced, and your weight issues will be addressed in lasting ways.

- When you read the Bible, you begin to know how to truly live.

- Find the best time to read your Bible each day and practice it daily until you wouldn't want to start your day without hearing from God. Try to find a time when there is a minimum amount of distraction; but you don't have to make it a huge chunk of time.

• It doesn't matter if you've seldom—or never—read the Bible. Start reading today.

Chapter 7

Digging Deeper

One of my best friends in the entire world sits in the office next to mine. We're blessed to see each other every day.

Pat Lewis has been my executive secretary for the past 13 years. She is someone who knows me inside and out. Years ago, Pat was instrumental in the wholehearted surrender of my life to the Lord. She was with me during the death of my daughter; the loss of my son's house in a fire; and when the news came that my husband, Johnny, had cancer. We've also had a lot of good times together—we've spent holidays at each other's houses, shopped together and gone for lunch, and we've welcomed each other's grandchildren into the world with joy.

Ask me why Pat and I are so close and I'd give you the same list of reasons why any two friends are: We share a commitment to seeing each other through thick and thin; we have similar likes and dislikes; we have an ease of communication; and we have a loyalty and pledge to each other's well-being.

I'd have to say that one of the strongest ties we have is the amount of time we've spent together. It's not as if we're inseparable—we do live our own lives! But we have an unspoken pledge to go deep into each other's lives. And that trust has only developed over time. It's one of the reasons we're such good friends today.

How about you? What is your best friend like? Chances are good that you've come to know your best friend over the years because you've invested quality time together.

The same thing is true with your spiritual life.

Have you ever sat in church and felt like an outsider when it came to your relationship with the Lord? Maybe the church was having a time of corporate prayer; all around you were people who were fervently talking to God, but you wondered what all the intensity was about.

Or maybe you've listened to someone talk about a relationship with the Lord, and that person mentions God with a closeness you're unfamiliar with.

Or perhaps you've sung worship songs with phrases such as "You're all I want—you're all I need" or "I'm desperate for You, Jesus," and you have to ask if you're sincerely singing those phrases, because in your most honest moments you're not sure if you are.

What does it truly mean to know Jesus Christ—to know what He's like or not like? Have you been able to point to some experience in your life and say, "Jesus was so real to me then . . . and I can tell you He's just as real to me today"?

One of the keys to knowing Christ is similar to knowing any good friend. You're invited to spend time with that person, to go deep with him or her, and vice versa. You're invited not to sip, but to drink deeply from a relationship that offers you something more than just a passing acquaintance. You're invited to "do life" together in real communion.

How does this happen with the Lord?

One of the primary ways is found in studying the Bible. I'm not talking about reading the Bible every day as we focused on in the last chapter. I'm talking about regularly digging in to what the Lord says about Himself and the plan He has for you as found in the pages of Scripture.

This is an invitation you don't want to miss.

When you study the Bible—when you open it up and mine the depths of its contents—you will find a depth of living you won't find anywhere else. This depth is crucial for the balance that's so necessary in your life. When you truly know who the Lord is, you will fall in love with the God of wonders; and the rest of your life has the opportunity to fall into place.

No Casual Conversations

What does studying the Bible possibly have to do with losing weight? Much more than you might think. Weight loss is not just a physical issue; it's also a spiritual issue. True change starts when you begin to ingest truth into your life, and God is the ultimate source of all truth.

Remember also that lasting change happens when you make a series of small, positive choices, day after day. Studying the Bible is part of each week's First Place 4 Health meeting. You're also invited to work through a few pages of a Bible study book each day, on your own, in preparation for that week's meeting. It takes only about 10 to 15 minutes per day.

The idea of studying the Bible may be completely new to you. Maybe you've never considered yourself a student, and the idea of digging into a book throws you off. Or maybe the Bible has always confounded you—it just seems too complicated. Perhaps you've never known how truly eye-opening a Bible study can be.

But consider for a moment what happens when you *don't* study the Bible. There are at least three dangers.

Lack of Knowledge Affects the Truth

When you don't study the Bible to understand what it truly says, chances are that you will make the Bible say anything you want it to say. That's dangerous.

But when you open your Bible and study it, you have the opportunity to know what Bible passages really mean. You can see for yourself what Scripture says in the context in which it was written. "Context" takes into account the specific background and circumstances of a passage. It gives you a correct framework for knowing what a particular passage is talking about.

For instance, some portions of Scripture were written to a specific group of people during a specific time in history. Other portions were written poetically or metaphorically, like when Psalm 57:1 talks about how we can take refuge in the shadow of God's *wing*—it's not that God is an actual bird; rather, this is an image of God's protection.

There's a sort of darkly funny story about a man who was flipping through his Bible one day, looking for a specific word from the Lord to apply to his life. He flipped to one passage that said, "Judas went out and hanged himself," and then flipped to another that said, "Go thou and do likewise," and then a third that said, "What you are about to do, do quickly."

That story is probably just an old joke told by preachers, but it illustrates connecting three portions of Scripture that have nothing to do with one another. When Scripture is applied out of context, the results can be unhealthy, even harmful. Entire false religions have been based on improper study, interpretation and application of the Bible.

An example of a verse that could be wrongly interpreted is 1 Peter 3:7, unless the entire passage surrounding the verse is studied carefully. Consider this scenario: You're reading your Bible one day and you quickly read 1 Peter 3:7, noticing that it calls women "weaker partner." So you think to yourself that if the Bible teaches that women are weak, then you shouldn't exercise very much, or perhaps you shouldn't lift weights or do strength training.

What 1 Peter 3:7 really says is this:

Husbands, in the same way be considerate as you live with your wives, and treat them with respect as the weaker partner and as heirs with you of the gracious gift of life, so that nothing will hinder your prayers.

There is so much truth to unpack in this one verse that entire sermons have been preached on it. This verse is actually an instruction to husbands to be considerate toward their wives. When you look at other Bible translations, it becomes clear that the idea behind "weaker partner" is closer to "precious vessel." Peter instructs husbands to live with their wives as if they were "valuable vases," and to be considerate and caring toward them. It's a positive verse for women, not a negative one, and by no means does it imply that women should not exercise or do strength training!

Lack of Knowledge Affects Knowing Christ

Ask people—even those who have received Jesus as their Savior—what their favorite portion of Scripture is, and you might hear some strange replies.

- Oh, uh . . . you know . . . that whole "love your neighbor" thing.

- Uh . . . *God helps those who help themselves*—that's in the Bible isn't it? (It's not in the Bible, by the way.)

- John 3:16—can't quote it, but you sure see it sometimes on signs in sports arenas.

You see, it's far easier to call yourself a Christian than to follow Christ. To truly know His words and what He's like, you need to spend time with Him, just as you would spend time with anyone who is a good friend.

When you don't study Scripture, you miss out. It's much harder to know the depth and substance of what you truly say you believe. Christ is known when you spend time with Him; it's that much harder to know Him when you don't know anything about Him.

Think of studying Scripture as your conversation with God. It's not casual conversation; it's the full-meal deal. It's where you sit down and explore who Jesus Christ is and the pathway He invites you to walk.

Lack of Knowledge Affects Getting Healthy

When you don't study Scripture, life transformation can still happen, but it happens at a slower pace. You get snippets of Scripture from daily reading, but studying Scripture gets you to the heart and core of the matter.

Studying the Bible on your own throughout the week and with a group once a week helps you understand the Word of God so that you can apply it to your life. The First Place 4 Health topical Bible studies directly relate to issues that all of us go through. The studies are targeted to areas in which we all struggle.

For example, we might have a study on resisting temptation, and in that study we look closely at the words of 1 Corinthians 10:13:

No temptation has seized you except what is common to man. And God is faithful, he will not let you be tempted beyond what you can bear. But when you are tempted, he will also provide a way out so that you can stand up under it.

What will this verse look like in your life? How will it apply to weight loss? What will it look like in your life the next time you're feeling down and you head to the refrigerator to pick yourself back up?

Those are the questions we'll walk through together in a Bible study. Our Bible studies take Scripture and apply it to life.

One woman in my group was in her early 70s when her husband died. She had gone to a Catholic school as a girl and had been raised in the church but never really studied the Bible. She told me that once she began to study the Bible, she felt like she never wanted to stop. She had found an oasis. You could actually see the peace that came over her when she began studying the Bible on a regular basis.

A Key Part of the Plan for Success

Why study the Bible? There is no simpler answer than "Because it's good for you and leads to balance in life." Studying the Bible regularly is one of the small choices you can make day after day that leads to lasting success.

In 2 Timothy 2:15, the Bible gives us a clear picture of what it looks like to study the Bible:

Do your best to present yourself to God as one approved, a workman who does not need to be ashamed and who correctly handles the word of truth.

Correctly handling the word of truth is what having a regular Bible study is all about.

Your invitation to have a regular Bible study is closely linked with reading Scripture every day. But they are not exactly the same. The First Place 4 Health distinction is that in addition to reading the Bible, you study a specific area of the Bible for an entire week and use discussion questions to help you learn what the text means. Each day in the study you are provided a few questions to work through and answer.

Each First Place 4 Health Bible study book contains 10 weeks of study. Each week has 5 days of questions related to the Scriptures you are studying. Days 6 and 7 are reserved for prayer and for reflection on what you have learned that week and applied.

The Components of Bible Study

One lifelong healthy practice is to learn how to study the Bible on your own. Essentially, Bible study breaks down into three components: observation, interpretation and application.

Observation

Observation simply means looking at the text. When you sit down to study Scripture, read through the passage several times. Don't jump to conclusions right away; just look to see what's happening in the passage. Imagine you're a newspaper reporter asking these questions: Who's talking? Who's listening? Where is this taking place? What's going on? When did this happen?

Interpretation

Interpretation means that you correctly determine the meaning of a particular passage. There are a variety of criteria for determining this, but here are three good rules of thumb:

1. *Interpret a passage grammatically and historically.* For example, you will read a psalm similar to how you'd read a poem, noting any play on words or word emphasis and any metaphors. You will read the book of Acts as history—these events happened in a specific place and time.

2. *Interpret a passage in its context.* Look at the rest of the chapter, or chapters, surrounding the passage you're seeking to

interpret. What does the passage you want to interpret mean within the flow of the book?

3. *Interpret a passage in light of the rest of Scripture.* Compare verses with other verses in other books of the Bible. There is a marvelous harmony within the Bible.

Application

Application is when you apply to your life what you've learned from the observation and interpretation stages. It's when you ask, How will my life be different if I apply what Scripture says in this passage?

You may also want to use some additional resources outside of the First Place 4 Health studies. The following resources will enhance your study time in God's Word. You may want to acquire these various resources over a period of time.

Different Translations

Choose a Bible translation that you enjoy using. Some of us grew up hearing the *King James Version,* but there are also many excellent modern translations, such as the *New International Version,* the *English Standard Version,* the *New Century Version,* the *New Living* translation or the *New American Standard. The Message* Bible by Eugene Peterson is also a creative and moving modern paraphrase—it was translated from the original languages concept by concept rather than word by word. My recommendation is to enjoy reading the paraphrases, such as *The Message* or the *Living Bible,* but to study from one of the word-by-word translations.

Spend some time in a local Christian bookstore and read some familiar passages in different versions, then select the one that speaks to your heart. Each First Place 4 Health Bible study is written for use with the *New International Version.* You can use another translation, although it might make answering the Bible study questions slightly more difficult.

A Parallel Bible

This type of Bible includes two to four translations right next to each other in columns. When you study God's Word, it is often useful to read several different translations because each one gives a different insight into each verse.

A Concordance

This book contains an alphabetized list of all the words from the Bible. If you can just remember a part of a verse, but you don't know where it's found, you can look up just one main word from that verse in a concordance and find the verse. A concordance will also help you study different topics or words from the Bible.

Bible Commentaries

Bible commentaries are written by scholars to explain passages and to provide a broader understanding of a Bible passage. There are a wide variety of commentaries available, either in a single volume for the entire Bible or in multiple volumes for each book of the Bible.

I recommend *The Bible Knowledge Commentary* by John F. Walvoord and Roy B. Zuck, two scholars from Dallas Theological Seminary. This excellent two-volume set will help you get to the meaning of the text without any complicated jargon.

A Bible Dictionary

This reference tool will give you insight into the cultural background of the Bible and help you understand definitions of difficult terms like "atonement" and "sanctification."

A Study Bible

As an alternative to several of these resources, consider buying a good study Bible. Like the variety of Bible translations, there are many different study Bibles available. Visit your local Christian bookstore and look through the various types of study Bibles. Talk with a salesperson to make an informed decision. I recommend the *Life Application Study Bible (New International Version)* as a very good, practical resource.

Bible Study Software

Almost anything in print today can also be found in an electronic version, either through a publisher or online. One excellent resource is E Sword (www.e-sword.net), which offers a variety of Bible versions, commentaries, dictionaries, and study notes—all for free.

Another good website is provided by the International Bible Society (www.ibs.org). This site offers online Bibles and search tools, as well as summaries and study helps.

Bible Gateway offers concordances, study helps and search tools. Find them at www.biblegateway.com

Your Plan Today

Studying Scripture may be a new idea to you. Within your specific goal to lose weight, it may be the farthest thing from your mind. But as you begin to dig deeply into God's Word and study what you read, many new insights about God will jump from the pages into your mind and heart. These insights will, in turn, help you live a balanced life filled with lasting wholeness and health.

Whenever I see people who are studying the Bible every day and then talking about what they're learning for 30 minutes together at class each week, I see God's Word working in their lives in profound ways.

Checklist for Success

- Life change happens when you begin to ingest truth. It is God who is the ultimate source of all truth. With the truth of His Word in your life, different areas of your life will come into balance, and weight issues will be addressed in lasting ways.

- Studying the Bible is different from simply reading it. Both reading and study are important. Reading the Bible is like a snack; but studying the Bible is a full meal.

- First Place 4 Health offers Bible study books that help you. They take about 10 to 15 minutes per day to work through, and 30 minutes to discuss each week at your First Place 4 Health meeting.

- It doesn't matter if you've never studied the Bible. You can start today.

First Place 4 Health in Real Life

Heidi McGraw
Montgomery, Minnesota

I heard a doctor from California share on a Christian radio station about the change God had brought to his life regarding weight loss. He said that what it boiled down to was his lack of obedience to God and that he was not taking care of his temple (body), in which the Holy Spirit dwelled. This hit me hard.

As a mother of three, I knew how important it is that my children obey me, yet my life was an example of disobedience to the God of the Universe. I knew that I needed to do something about it, because I hated how I looked; I lived with guilt every time I ate, and it was a self-defeating cycle. I'm sad and embarrassed to say that I remember looking at my beautiful teenage daughter with intense envy because she was beautiful, and I only had memories of being like her now that my body was in disrepair.

I talked with a friend, and we decided to keep each other accountable and to encourage each another. After a very short time, I realized that I didn't know where or how to begin. I understood the concept but lacked the plan to follow through.

In the fall of 2005, I noticed that one of the ladies from our church was losing weight. When I asked her what she was doing, she said it was a biblical weight-loss program called First Place. After about six people asked her what she was doing, she decided that perhaps she should lead a group for our church. She gathered names of interested people and teamed up with another lady who was currently following the plan with her. Thus the First Place 4 Health program was started at our church.

We began meeting on March 18, 2006, a day that will be forever etched in my memory. I was so ready, and my heart was softened to do whatever God called me to do. I embraced the program and took it very seriously. I started walking four or more times each week, ate within my guidelines and, for the first time in my life, spent time daily in God's Word. I had become a Christian in the spring of 1998, but I lacked growth in my relationship with Christ. I was always too busy to take time for God on a daily basis, and I missed out on a deeper relationship with Him for many years.

My motive in joining First Place was to lose weight; but once I was part of the Bible study, God took hold of my heart and life. Although my before-and-after pictures reveal a significant change, they will never reveal the greatness of my inner heart change. Scripture memorization has been such a blessing. As I go through trials, I remind myself of God's truth, and I know that His plan is always for my good and to build my character. The deep relationship I have built with my sisters in Christ has been awesome as well.

First Place 4 Health teaches that balancing the four aspects of life is so important because we are to be imitators of Christ, and He grew in all of these areas (see Luke 2:51-52). My relationship with Christ my Savior is my foremost concern each day, and I delight in taking care of my body to honor Him.

Since I have lost 63 pounds, I have had so many opportunities to share what a difference Christ has made in my life, and I give Him all the glory. I have so much energy, and I love that I can live each day without the guilt and stronghold that Satan once held over me. My days are filled with thoughts of the Lord, and I sing praises from deep within me because He rescued me from my muddy pit.

Before	After

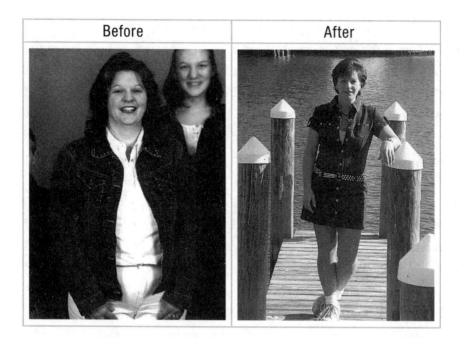

My family members have witnessed my health journey and have changed how they eat as well, seeking what God desires for us all. I have led a First Place for Youth study with the senior high girls of our church because I believe that if we can teach our younger generation what God's design and purpose is for us, they can enjoy a lifetime of living for Him and not waste years as I did.

Thank you, First Place 4 Health, for obeying what God has called you to do—help bring about a change in people's lives for His glory. Words will never adequately express what my heart knows or feels.

Jennifer Krogh
Kewaunee, Wisconsin

What an awesome God we serve! As I reflect on the past 15 years and where God has brought the obese woman shown in my before picture, I am still in awe.

The "before" picture is me at my heaviest, with my first child, Nathaniel. I didn't know the Lord as my Savior then, but God used the pregnancy and birth of my children to speak to my heart. I realized that I wanted to be a success as a mom because of so many years filled with rebellion, guilt and failure. I wanted to do this parent thing right. The birth of my children also brought me back to church, a place I had avoided since my freshman year of high school. I knew it was important for my children to be brought up attending Sunday School and church in order to make a decision to follow Christ for themselves someday. When my sons were toddlers, the Holy Spirit convicted my heart and I received Christ as my savior in September 1988.

In December 1992, I was looking through a Christian catalog and saw a Christ-centered weight-loss program advertised (not First Place). I highlighted and circled the item and told my husband this was all I wanted for Christmas, but I didn't want him to tell anyone else. I had a huge fear of failure. In the past, I had tried diet pills, various weight-loss

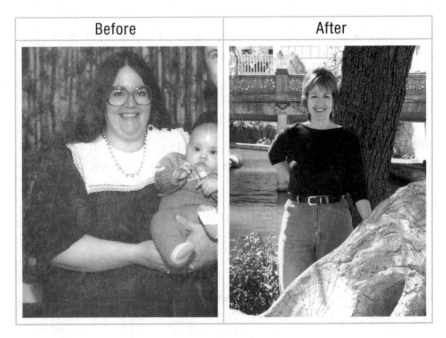

Before	After

programs, and starvation. I was not going to attempt another diet program until I knew how to bring Christ into it. On January 4, 1993, I began the weight-loss program at home with only a few people aware of what I was doing.

One of those people was our pastor's wife. Although Cindy was fit, she had to work at it, so I felt safe in telling her. She was at a women's luncheon where someone expressed a desire for a Christian weight-management support group. She called me when she got home and said, "What about leading a group here at church?" My first reaction was, *No way!* I thought I couldn't start a group unless I was at my goal weight. The Lord threw that excuse out immediately. On March 15, 1993, I stood (shaking) in front of our first group—leading by the grace of God. I was the heaviest one in the group.

That first year I lost 80 pounds. I led the group for the next eight-and-a-half years. I lost a bit more and fluctuated during some stressful times, but I never gained back all the weight, as I had always done before. This was the first time I had ever lost weight and kept it off.

In 1998, a woman joined our group who had lived in Singapore. She had been a member of a First Place group for five years. Judy had a history miraculously similar to mine. Needless to say, we understood each other. She enthusiastically shared First Place with me. My response was polite, but I wasn't interested. However, God's timing is perfect. In the summer of 2001, I was ordering some materials online, and while browsing the site, I came across a book called *First Place*. I purchased the book, intending to supplement the lessons for our group. The title sounded familiar, and I asked Judy if it was the same as her old program. It was. When I read the book, my excitement grew.

I prayed and asked Judy to pray about doing First Place together. We began the Bible study in October 2001. We met each week, exchanged CRs (commitment records), and became familiar with the program. I had never reached my goal weight in all those years in the other program.

I knew that my successes were greater than a number on the scale, but I still wanted to reach that goal. On December 17, the same day First Place was officially ushered in, I reached my goal! To me, it was no coincidence that these two events occurred on the same day. I believe it was another confirmation from the Lord that, yes, this is the way; walk in it.

Our First Place 4 Health group began in Kewaunee on January 14, 2002. In that first year, the Lord brought many others from outside our community, some traveling from as far away as 100 miles one way. These individuals wanted to take the First Place program back to their communities. In the fall of 2002, I attended the First Place Focus Week, and it was there that I knew I was to step out as a Networking Leader for my state. It was also at Focus Week that I wholeheartedly completed memorizing Psalm 139, something I had attempted many times but never followed through on. Scripture memorization is now an important part of the balanced life for me.

In my 20s, I made several unhealthy attempts to reach what appeared to be an impossible weight-loss goal. I only managed to tag that goal and then regain the weight rapidly, becoming heavier than when I started. In 2006, the Lord equipped me to achieve the goal that I had always thought unrealistic and impossible. I believe it is because of His goodness and the blessing of obedience. It has taken many years to get to this place. It has been work, and it has been a process; but it has been worth more than I can express. Thank You, Lord, for First Place 4 Health!

Karrie Smyth
Brandon, Manitoba, Canada

My family loves to eat! Whether happy or sad, if we're together, you can bet that food is there. For the first 30 years of my life, I didn't realize that I had a problem with food. I was active enough to compensate for

Before	After

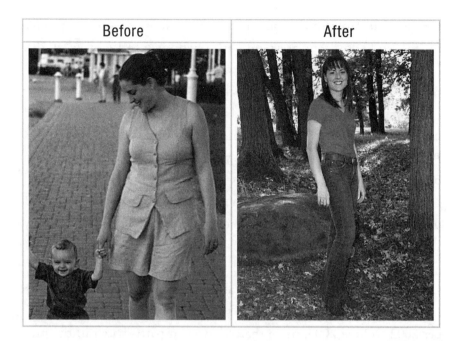

what I ate. But after having two children, I found myself incapable of losing the weight I had gained. I tried a number of different diets with little success. I knew what to do but couldn't seem to do it. With the pressures of work, being a wife and mother, and a daughter whose dad was dying of cancer, life was out of control, and so was my eating.

In the spring of 2002, during a simulcast, Carole Lewis shared how God had proved Himself faithful to her even through the tragic death of her daughter Shari on Thanksgiving Day 2001. I was struck by the fact that this woman—an author, speaker, wife, mother and grandmother—could have such balance in her life in the midst of such tragedy! I needed what she had! So, the next day I bought every First Place book I could find. I began reading the First Place Bible study *Life Under Control* and devoured every page!

Though I had been a Christian for most of my life, I had allowed the Lord to have very little control of my life. I learned more and more about the Lord and His great love for me. I learned that my body is the temple of the Holy Spirit who is in me, and that Jesus paid a huge price for me, so I should honor God with my body (see 1 Cor. 6:19-20). I poured all the willpower I had into studying the Bible, and God faithfully provided the self-control to eat well and exercise.

It was clear that I was addicted to sugar and that turning to food instead of turning to God robbed Him of the opportunity to bless me. Praise the Lord, a transformation was taking place in my heart and body. My hunger for food was being replaced by a hunger for the Word of God, and it showed. By September 2002, I had lost more than 35 pounds, and my new body was a mere bonus compared to the intimacy I had found with the Lord.

People noticed the change and wanted the same thing for themselves. I started a First Place group at my church, and we couldn't keep up with the number of people who wanted to take part. From September 2002 to June 2005, more than 90 women participated in the program, and we collectively lost more than 1,000 pounds! God is so good!

In August 2005, my dad passed away. I allowed myself to return to old habits. I was angry with God. Though I was still leading a First Place group, I put on 17 pounds that year. The rising number on the scale wasn't enough to catch my attention; but praise God, He broke through to me! God is big enough to handle our anger, disappointments, grief and sorrows! He proved that in the good times and in the bad, He is still faithful! He blesses every humble step we take in obedience to Him. I returned to treating my body as the temple it is and the Lord helped me leave behind those 17 pounds.

In the midst of all of this, through many tests, I was diagnosed with Crohn's disease. Life with Crohn's means living with constant pain and discomfort. There is no known cure for Crohn's. On good days, I couldn't sit with my arms crossed due to the pressure this placed on my abdomen. On the bad days, I lay in bed unable to find relief. I lost all energy and often struggled to walk up and down stairs.

Whether because the Lord had chosen not to heal my dad or that I somehow thought I deserved Crohn's as punishment for years of abusing my body, I realized that I had never asked God to heal me. On February 19, 2007, I was marveling at all the Lord had done for me—overwhelmed that Jesus would die to pay the price for my sins and set me free from my burdens and oppression. How do you respond to a gift like that but accept it? I would gladly accept the healing of my body upon entrance to heaven, so why wouldn't I accept it before then? With feelings of fear as well as anticipation, I began asking Him for healing.

When we started a vacation on June 30, 2007, I was sick. Would I ever be able to keep up with my family as I once had? On July 2, while having more tests to determine the extent of the inflammation from Crohn's, the doctor asked me why I was there and what tests had been used in the diagnosis. I gave him the whole list. He asked where the Crohn's was located. I told him the area all the other tests had pinpointed. He turned the monitor around so that I could see. There was nothing there!

I had just been sick two days before. I nearly asked the Lord aloud what He was up to! Excitement started to pulse in me. Was I being healed? The next day, I woke to notice that I had no pain or discomfort. With an unspoken question to the Lord, I quit my medication and inwardly said, *Let's just see.* Praise the Lord, He can work with faith as small as a mustard seed! No pain returned!

My doctor cannot explain it. Not only is there no inflammation now, but there is also no sign of the damage that once was there! "The Mighty One has done great things for me—holy is His Name" (Luke 1:49).

God has shouldered my grief, bound up my broken heart, healed my body and set me free.

PART 3

Mind:
Seeking Balance Mentally

You might be wondering why there is only one chapter in this section. At First Place 4 Health, we believe that *what you think affects how you act.* We also believe that when you get the Word of God into your mind, you receive the very thoughts of God, which forever change your life for your good and for His glory.

That's not to say that every issue that involves the mental processes gets solved by memorizing Scripture. Certainly there are clinical issues, challenges, traumas and diseases that require therapy, medication or even surgery to work through and resolve. But within the everyday framework of life, Scripture addresses most of the issues we face.

You have read this before, but it bears repeating: Change starts when you begin to ingest truth in your life; and God is the ultimate source of all truth. With Him in your life, every area of life can come into balance.

Your invitation in this chapter is to make Scripture memory a regular part of your journey toward living that balanced life.

Chapter 8

Bible Thinking

A woman in my First Place 4 Health group recently became a leader in the program. Previously, whenever she showed up to class, she usually dressed in sweat pants and a T-shirt. Her attitude and demeanor were mirrored in her clothes. When she became a leader, her thinking began to change. She phoned me not long ago.

"Carole, you'll never guess what," she said. "I was reading in the leader's guide about how we're supposed to look nice whenever we lead a group. So I went out and got my hair cut and had the gray taken out, and I bought some new clothes. The people in my class hardly recognize me now."

I can't wait to see this woman again! People who have seen her say that she has a different countenance and carries herself in a more confident way. There is a spring in her step that hasn't been there before. She believes that she can lead the group, and she's choosing to look the part and take pride in her appearance as a leader. How wonderful!

My point is not that she changed her outward appearance but that she changed her thinking; and her thinking was what changed her behavior. How a person thinks affects how a person acts. Do you believe that? Proverbs 23:7 (*KJV*) tells us that as a man thinks in his heart, so is he (see also Prov. 27:19; Luke 6:45).

You see, God doesn't pry your fingers open and snatch away those things that you think are so important. He gently begins to replace them with what is of greater significance. He begins to work on your mind and heart and gently shows you a healthier way to live. Through this process of achieving mental balance, you begin to see that He has a better plan for your life.

The key is to allow God to fill your mind with thoughts that will enable you to grow. When this happens, you will find yourself changing not only in the way you think, but in all other areas of your life as well—physically, emotionally and spiritually. Changing your thinking is a gradual process; but as you begin to think in a new way, you will find that the Lord brings a new balance to your life that you've never experienced before.

Changing your thinking is vital to living a balanced life. The problem is, we all tend to like our old way of thinking.

The Dangerous Self-Talk in Our Head

What negative mental tapes are spinning around in your head? Those tapes might have been created from any number of sources—former teachers who said you weren't living up to your full potential; a parent who consistently told you that you were clumsy or stupid; someone at church who insisted that you weren't being spiritual enough or that God was upset with you; a well-meaning friend who left trauma in your life.

Your self-talk often springs from an effort to protect yourself. Self-talk tapes can rule your mind, shape your thoughts, form how you act and dictate the decisions you make. Sometimes you're not even aware that the tapes are playing. And if you are aware of the tapes, although you might realize that their messages are unhealthy, at least they are familiar—they are all you know. We often feel a false sense of security in whatever is familiar.

What does a self-talk tape sound like?

Suppose the phone rings, and it's someone from your church asking you to help out in some way. What's the first thing that comes to your mind?

- Yes, I need to help out. I always help out. That's what I do.

- No way am I going to help out. I always seem to get burned at church. I need to say no to protect myself.

- I can't do what's being asked of me. I'm not good at anything. I'm never good at anything.

If the first tape is the one that plays, those words will probably lead to stress, anxiety and burnout. If the second tape plays, it will lead to disillusionment or friendlessness; and if the third tape plays, it will lead to boredom, apathy and lost opportunities.

Your self-talk tapes tend to play whenever opportunities, crises or decisions come your way. You search your mind to see what you think is true, and then you act on whatever those tapes tell you to do. Self-talk leads to ingrained patterns of action. For good or bad, self-talk leads you to do what you've always done.

Certainly outside influences can affect you; yet the core truth is that what happens in your mind—what you tell yourself—leads to your behavior.

I used to work with a girl who was convinced that her husband was going to leave her. That was her mental tape, and it affected virtually every area of her life. She was a fearful person—everyone in the office felt it. The problem wasn't her husband—he seemed like a really nice guy. The problem was that her parents had divorced when she was young, and she had ingested a lot of hurt and insecurity in her past. Those experiences led to her mental tape that her husband would leave her.

On any Monday morning, if I asked this girl about her weekend, without fail she would tell me that something horrible had happened between her and her husband. I'd listen to her story, but none sounded as bad as this girl made it out to be. But that's not what she was telling herself. Her mind wouldn't allow her to see the good that truly existed in her marriage.

Another person I knew used to repeat this phrase: "Nobody gets a second chance to hurt me." This woman knew the Lord, and she knew what He says in His Word about forgiveness. It didn't matter to her. Somewhere in her past, she had been deeply hurt. As a protective layer, she saw her world only through the mental tape that she had convinced herself was true—she would never let anyone hurt her again.

Believing and saying "Nobody gets a second chance to hurt me" only hurt her. It's tough to be friends with a person who won't give you any room to make mistakes. Everyone who interacted with her felt as if they needed to walk on eggshells. If someone hurt her, in even the slightest way, her mental tape would kick in and she would give that person the cold shoulder from then on. It made her a very tough person to be friends with.

A man I know has never been able to please his mother. No matter what he does, it is never right. If he buys her a beautiful purse, she asks why he spent so much money. Even today, as a grown man, the words of his mother continue to hurt him so much that he says, "I can hear what she will say, or what she would say, if she knew, about any decision I make." Because of the critical nature of his mother, he is extremely critical of himself. He pushes himself to perfection because of the tape playing in his head of his mother's voice.

Faulty thinking can be horribly harmful. What goes on in our head eventually works its way out through our body. Our life is affected by what we think. And that's the problem if what's in our head is not the truth.

A Continual Feast

How do you get truth into your mind and play positive mental tapes? Simple: You take into your mind what God says is true. You ingest

Scripture. You memorize portions of God's Word. The words of Philippians 4:8 are so true for our lives:

> Finally brothers, whatever is true, whatever is noble, whatever is right, whatever is pure, whatever is lovely, whatever is admirable— if anything is excellent or praiseworthy—think about such things.

In memorizing the Word of God, your mind is shaped by the righteous Lord of the universe. Once you know what God's Word says, you're accountable to it. God has the answer in His Word for every situation in which you might find yourself, and His Word changes the way you think about those situations.

Consider the following two examples.

When someone doesn't have God's Word in his or her life, and that person does something stupid (we all make mistakes from time to time), what might that person say inwardly?

- I'm such an idiot.
- I can't do anything right.
- I'll never amount to anything. Might as well not even try.

Do you see how harmful self-talk can be? But when you have the Word of God in your mind, and you do something stupid (it's happened to me, that's for sure), what might you say to yourself? *You know, what I did right now is just not like me. But that doesn't mean that I'm dumb or stupid. I just made a mistake, and now I need to see if I can remedy that mistake. What verses come to mind right now to remind me of my identity in Christ? What does God say about me?*

Then you repeat to yourself any of the wonderful promises in Scripture that show your worth because of Christ. Isaiah 49:16 says that God loves us so much that He tells us, "I have engraved you on the palms of my hands." Jeremiah 31:3 describes God's love for His people as "an everlasting love." In 1 Peter 2:9, we see that we are "a chosen people, a royal priesthood, a holy nation, a people belonging to God, that [we] may declare the praises of Him."

When you immerse your mind in God's truth—His Word—His truth becomes the standard and criteria for how you think and act. You no longer make decisions on faulty self-talk but on something that's good and beneficial.

My friend Nancy Taylor discovered a verse that has revolutionized her attitude toward life: "All the days of the afflicted are bad, but a cheerful heart has a continual feast" (Prov. 15:15, *NASB*).

This is Nancy's story, in her own words, about applying what she knew to be true.

The week I was memorizing and meditating on Proverbs 15:15, I was set to fly to California for a workshop. The morning my plane was to depart, I arrived at the airport two hours early due to all the extra security. I checked my bags and went through the security line with ease. It was going to be a great day.

Shortly after this thought went through my mind, I was greeted at my gate with the word "Cancelled" flashing at the check-in desk. The waiting area sat eerily vacant, and my first instinct was to panic and convince myself that it was going to be a really bad day.

But the Holy Spirit tapped me on the shoulder, and the words of Proverbs 15:15 swept through my mind: "All the days of the afflicted are bad, but a cheerful heart has a continual feast."

I laughed out loud and then looked around to see if anyone had observed me. God was up to something. He was calling me to test His Word and see if it was true.

So, I took the challenge and set out to prove His Word.

At that moment I chose to have a cheerful heart and looked to see what "feast" might await me.

After standing in a long line for about 30 minutes, I discovered that all flights to Dallas had been canceled due to bad weather. My itinerary had called for a stopover in Dallas and then on to Oakland. When I stepped up to the counter, I greeted the clerk with a smile. She said, "I'm sorry, there is a flight available, but you will have to change airlines and you will be on a nonstop flight, arriving in Oakland two hours early."

My dimples deepened as I grinned even bigger and said to myself, *Continual feast!* I entered the airplane of my new flight and discovered that I had the entire row of seats to myself. I was able to read, study and rest for the entire three-hour flight. Quite a feast indeed!

I had tried God's Word, chosen to obey its truth and found it to be true. People can choose to be afflicted or cheerful—it's a choice.

Negative attitudes are contagious and will spread like a cancer in your life if left unchecked. By choosing to believe God's Word and live it through a positive attitude, a continual feast awaits us!

Nancy's story says it all. Second Peter 1:3 tells us that God gives us everything we need for life and godliness through *our knowledge of Him.*

How do you obtain knowledge of Him? Through knowledge of His Word.

Whenever your negative self-talk convinces you that you're worthless or stupid or unable do something to improve your health, it's as if you're saying that God doesn't have the power to make you into the person He wants you to be.

The Word of God will change the way you think about that.

Safety in the Night

When you've memorized Scripture, and you're facing a challenge that you can't see your way out of, or you're tempted to give up or give in to fear and discouragement, God will bring to mind Scripture that corresponds to your situation. He will give you strength for the road ahead.

I'm convinced that memorizing God's Word is a huge part of living a balanced life. We've got to start thinking in a healthy way—and we do that by filling our mind with the very thoughts of God.

It's easy for me to resort to sad thoughts when I think about my three grandchildren whose mother is in heaven. Our son-in-law Jeff is a wonderful father to those girls—Cara, Christen and Amanda—but he's not a mother. Never claims to be. So occasionally I wake up in the middle of the night and begin to think "mama thoughts" about these kids.

Cara is married to a wonderful man, Michael. When she became pregnant, they lived in Abilene, Texas, almost 350 miles from where Johnny and I live in Galveston Bay, yet I was determined to be there when she gave birth. We women need our mothers around, even when we're grown up!

About six weeks before the baby was due, Cara started going into labor. I made three trips to Abilene before their child was born. At times, I felt pushed toward anxious thoughts. But I was there when our first great-grandchild, the wonderful Luke Ryan Parker, arrived in early September, and I stayed at Cara and Michael's house for a week. Everything worked out in the end.

What got me through those times of anxiety leading up to the delivery? Or rather, what *replaced my anxiety*?

Scripture.

Whenever I woke up in the middle of the night, I'd ask the Lord to bring to mind Scripture that I had memorized. Sometimes I'd wake up in the night singing Scripture memory songs—they're now so deep in my soul. Psalm 4:8 was a great comfort to me:

> I will lie down and sleep in peace,
> For you alone, O Lord
> Make me dwell in safety.

Instead of the old tape spinning in my head, God's Word spoke to me loud and clear. God was in control of everything, including Cara and Michael's baby. I could rest in the Lord, knowing that He is good all the time.

Memorizing Scripture is so beneficial for us. Psalm 107:20 shows a correlation between Scripture and healing:

> He sent forth his Word and healed them;
> he rescued them from the grave.

I'm not saying that we should avoid doctors or shun surgery or throw away our eyeglasses. But it makes sense that what goes into our mind eventually works its way out through our body.

There is a very strong mind-body connection. When we're embarrassed (something that happens in the mind), our faces turn red (something that happens to the body). When we're nervous (mind), we get butterflies in our stomach (body). If what's going on in our head is harmful, that's bound to affect our health in a negative way. Conversely, if what's going on in our head is the Word of God, that's equally bound to affect our health in a positive way.

But it's more than that. God, through His Word, is the only one who has the power to ultimately change us. Through the Holy Spirit, God applies His teaching—His Word—to our life. The older I get, the more I believe this. I have a good friend who laughs with me at all the good advice we've given that nobody has followed. These days my advice-giving activity is way down. Why bother? If advice comes only from me, it's easy to ignore. Now, if someone asks me for counsel, I always try to offer what God says. I want God's advice to permeate the person's mind.

What are you going through right now? And what does God say about that situation? Everything in the Bible has been given to us to help us live according to God's purposes. His Word is truth.

I Can't Memorize

When people hear that it's so beneficial to memorize Scripture, one response I often hear is, "I can't memorize Scripture. I've never been good at memorizing"—or some variation of this.

But just think about how many other things we memorize: phone numbers, addresses, jingles to television commercials, lyrics to songs. The mind is an incredible "computer" and can do much more than we typically give it credit for.

You *can* memorize Scripture, even if you've never done it before. It doesn't matter if it doesn't stick in your mind immediately. Just start where you are. The First Place 4 Health program isn't about doing all things perfectly all of the time. Beginning to choose positive changes, such as memorizing Scripture, is what we ask you to start incorporating into your life so that you will know what balance is all about.

I had convinced myself that I could never memorize Scripture, and I was resistant to even trying at first. But what made things a whole lot easier for me was the Scripture memory CDs (in the back of the First Place 4 Health Bible studies) that are set to up-tempo music. You can listen while you're driving or walking or working out. I like to listen to the Scripture CDs in the morning while I walk on a treadmill. (You can also download First Place 4 Health songs—one or several—online at iTunes.)

When you join a 12-week group session of First Place 4 Health, you are invited to learn 10 verses during that time (there is no verse memorization for the first two weeks) and to say your verse each week to your group leader when you weigh in. Often, group leaders will give prizes to members who can say all 10 verses at the end of the 12-week session. The goal is to get Scripture into your mind.

We also encourage you to seek accountability as you learn Scripture. It's a lot easier for me to work on verses each morning with my workout partner. We can say 10 verses in 3 minutes, because we practice saying them all the time. Permeating our minds with Scripture sets a positive tone for the entire day.

Balanced Thinking

We hear so many messages every day that are simply not true. But we have an oasis in God's Word, which helps us distinguish what is true. Even when we're not feeling happy, we can always have hope and joy in the Lord and His promises to us who believe in Him.

In many ways, Scripture memorization is a process—a learned skill. Typically, everything in life that changes you for the better is a learned skill—we learn to walk, we learn to eat right. And we learn to memorize Scripture. So, if the invitation to memorize Scripture feels daunting right now, just start where you are. Sometimes you have to step out of your comfort zone and say yes to a good thing. With God's help, you will be able to do what He calls you to do.

Begin to memorize God's Word, and you'll be that much closer to living a balanced life that leads to changes that are lasting and permanent.

Checklist for Success

- Weight loss begins in the mind.

- When you change your thoughts, you change how you live.

- Scripture memory changes your thoughts to align with God's thoughts.

- If you think you can't memorize Scripture, just give it a try. Use the First Place 4 Health Scripture memory CDs, or learn the verses with a friend.

First Place 4 Health in Real Life

Tammy Price
Myrtle Beach, South Carolina

In 1998, as a new bride, I wanted to look great for my husband. I asked God to help me lose weight. I expected Him to just zap it off. Instead, He chose to put a First Place book by Carole Lewis into my hands. At the time, I was unable to attend any meetings, but I consumed every word in the book. I read through it more than once and was so encouraged by all the success stories. I was especially encouraged by the fact that they (like me) had tried everything to lose weight and maintain some semblance of control and balance in life. My life was spinning out of control, especially when it came to my eating. As a new Christian, God was convicting me of my out-of-control lifestyle.

I read in John 10:10 that Jesus came to Earth so that we would have abundant life; but my life was miserable. I hated going places because of the way I looked. When I read Carole's book, I just knew this was the answer to my prayers. I was ready to experience life instead of dread it. Yet, I had no idea of the exceeding abundance God would bring to my life and how He would answer prayer!

At first I was overwhelmed at the thought of a lifestyle change and writing down everything I ate. Yet this activity taught me to rely on

God. I was amazed at the excitement God gave me to do this. Each morning, I got up a little earlier so that I could meet with Him in prayer and Scripture reading, and surrender my will and my day to Him. After a while, a few minutes with God were not enough, and I got up earlier and earlier with an overwhelming desire to meet with Him.

My desire to follow the program also grew while I shrank! I had been walking for some time, and my body was used to it, so I upped my fitness level challenge. I started jogging and finally quit smoking, which I had also tried to do a zillion times. The very first time I jogged, I lasted only 30 seconds. With a lot of prayer, I threw out my cigarettes. I couldn't run if I smoked. With asthma problems, I could barely breathe at times!

I committed it all to God on a daily basis and recited to myself as I jogged, "I can do all things through Christ who gives me strength" (Phil. 4:13). In about one month, I was running one to two miles a day, and my asthma actually went away! I lost 30 pounds in three months and went from a size 12 to a size 7!

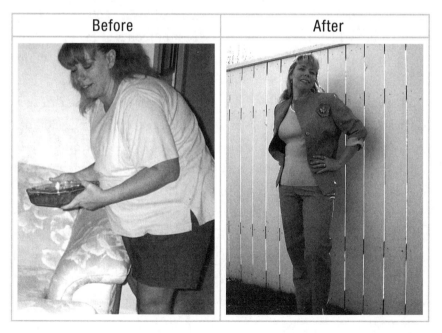

Before	After

Funny, one of the reasons I hadn't quit smoking before was that I was afraid I would gain weight. Through one of the memory verses during that first three months, I learned that my body is His temple, and along with unhealthy eating, I was defiling His temple with cigarettes. Through this struggle, God showed me that He will enable me to gain victory in any area that I need to bring into obedience to Him. He does the "doing" as long as we do the surrendering and abiding.

I wish I could say that I never had another struggle with food and exercise. But by the end of my fourth pregnancy, I weighed a high of 228, because I foolishly didn't stick with what I knew to do during those first three pregnancies. God has taught me that even when we aren't faithful, He is always ready to meet us in our place of need. He has brought me back to a lifestyle of freedom once again, and I'm back home at First Place 4 Health, even leading a group again—this time through an online ministry. So far my total weight loss is 70 pounds. My goal is no longer only to please my husband, but also to glorify God as He continues to help me toward my goal of losing 100 pounds. My spiritual growth, however, is by far the best outcome of my First Place 4 Health journey. I can't imagine where I'd be without this program, without this way of life and without my commitment to put God first!

Through my daily prayer time—being taught and trained to seek His heart, to journal my prayers and to encourage others daily, God has grown Hearts of Prayer Ministries, a nonprofit women's ministry in which I teach others the truths that God has taught me over these past few years. He has burdened my heart to equip and encourage others in prayer and holiness. He has also taken this once selfish and shy, too-fat-to-go-out-of-the-house lady and turned her into a Christian author and speaker who gets up in front of people and ministers to women all over the world! It is so humbling that God could take someone who was so hopeless and such a mess and use me to help others in the very same area!

The weight loss has been great, but the most incredible part has been my intimate, growing relationship with Almighty God. What He has done on the outside of me is just a fragment of what He is doing on the inside. He used my desire to lose weight to bring me to First Place and to help me seek Him. He is growing in me such a love for Him, for prayer and for His Word that I just can't get enough. As I allow Him daily to have all of me, He allows me to live out the verse "But seek first his kingdom and his righteousness, and all these things will be given to you as well" (Matt. 6:33). He is doing above and beyond all that I could dream, ask or imagine. What began as a physical need turned into spiritual transformation.

Karen Arnett
Evans, Georgia

In 1994, I found myself in the emergency room weighing 416 pounds. Having been overweight since the age of 4, I had been on many diets. I had lost as much as 65 pounds, several times, then always gained the weight back plus more. Diets didn't work because I used food to comfort myself and push down any anxiety I was feeling. I mostly overate from boredom. God used this emergency room medical scare to get my attention.

Feeling very vulnerable at this point, I found myself listening to an overweight nurse talk about a "fat-counter diet." I went home the next day and started counting every gram of fat I ate. In the next six months, I lost 68 pounds. I still overate at times, did not exercise, and I still had many of the bad eating habits I had developed over my lifetime.

In May 1995, a friend started the First Place program at our church. She encouraged me to come to orientation to see what the program was about. It was a stricter plan than what I was on, but I liked the spiritual aspect. I knew that I wasn't submitting this area of my life to God and that only He could truly help me overcome the bondage I was in. With the help and support of people who cared, I was able to commit myself wholeheartedly to God and follow the First Place program. Over the next two years, I lost 198 additional pounds, for a total of 266 pounds.

First Place helped me realize the reasons I was overeating. Through keeping an Awareness Record, I found that watching TV was a big problem for me. I ate while watching TV and didn't think about how much food I was consuming. And when I watched TV, I had a strong urge to eat. I stopped watching TV and rarely watch it now. First Place helped me make lifestyle changes that I keep to this day. Everything I learned in First Place I still do: I make healthy eating choices; I exercise; I put God first; and I seek His help in every struggle. I have learned to trust Him. He is faithful, and He calls us to faithfulness.

There is no quick fix out there. You can lose weight by eating a low-carb diet or having gastrointestinal bypass surgery, but if you don't learn

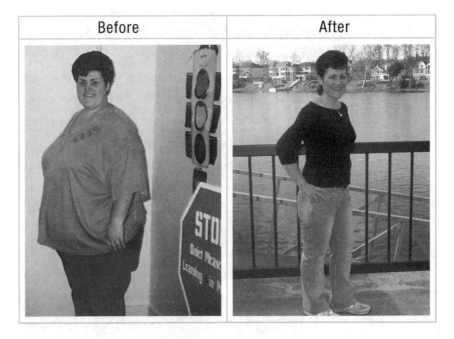

| Before | After |

to eat in a healthy way and exercise properly, you will most likely gain the weight back. First Place is something you can do for the rest of your life. As Carole Lewis tells us, "Maintenance on First Place is just more of First Place." Maintaining my weight is something I work at every day. Some days are easy and some are hard, but with God's strength and help, I am persevering.

It has been 12 years now, and I have lost a total of 271 pounds. An anthropologist from The National Weight Control Registry (the NWCR tracks people who have lost at least 30 pounds and maintained it for at least a year) interviewed me several years ago and conducted a personality survey. Her conclusion was that I needed the accountability that First Place offers.

I still need it, because I still have all the same tendencies I had before starting First Place. It is so wonderful to be in the hands of a loving God. He has been so good to me. My prayer is that He will continue to use me to help others see that He cares about every detail of our lives and that nothing is too hard for Him. Only in giving all of yourself to God can you have true victory in every area of your life.

Joy Bianchi
Chicago, Illinois

I can remember the first time I thought that I was fat. I was 8 or 10, and our family doctor told my mother that I was a little "husky." I have struggled with weight all of my life and experimented with a lot of different diets that worked temporarily or didn't work at all.

I have come to realize that God has given me this "thorn" for a purpose—His purpose. I had considered myself a strong, self-sufficient woman. Admitting defeat was tantamount to failure. I think that is why

God has chosen to reveal His power to me in my struggle with weight. It has been His outlet—the way that He truly could reveal His power to me—because it is a struggle I have never been able to overcome on my own.

About one year into the First Place program, I had learned a lot but was still fluctuating in my weight. In desperation, during a conversation with Ginny, an accountability partner from First Place, I let her know that I had been keeping a gastric bypass ad in my wallet for over a year. If First Place didn't work, surgery was my next step. Since then, I've learned to wait for God's timing. That night during that conversation with Ginny, I put my trust in God and His way for weight loss.

It's much easier for me to say what has changed in my life since following the precepts of First Place 4 Health than to define how it has happened; but I can tell you that I am a different person, and not just from the outside.

My Life Before First Place:

- I ate whatever, whenever, according to my lust for more.
- I didn't exercise.
- My only exercise was at a high level of stress.
- I would look at myself in the mirror and speak only words of hate to myself.
- I would "medicate" myself with food, not even realizing how infrequently I was eating out of true hunger.
- I was living a self-fulfilling prophecy of self-hate.
- I was using food in place of God for comfort and pleasure.
- I was at an uncomfortable and dangerous weight.
- I couldn't go 4 hours without food, let alone fast for a full 24 hours.
- My life was filled with self-indulgence.

My Life Since First Place:

- I eat with better, and God-honoring, motives.
- I exercise—I actually enjoy it! I used to dread having to run "the mile" in high school. Now I routinely do 3.1 miles (5K).
- I can look at myself in the mirror and see myself more as God sees me. I can also look in the mirror without speaking words of hate to myself.
- I am in the Word consistently and realize firsthand an immediate correlation between a daily quiet time with God and in-control living.
- I realize that I will always be dependent on God for help in this area and that I will probably always depend on others for love and support, as it has been so abundantly shown to me in First Place.
- I memorize Scripture and enjoy it.
- I have a First Place accountability partner who promised me that she would be my partner until my weight came off. She is now

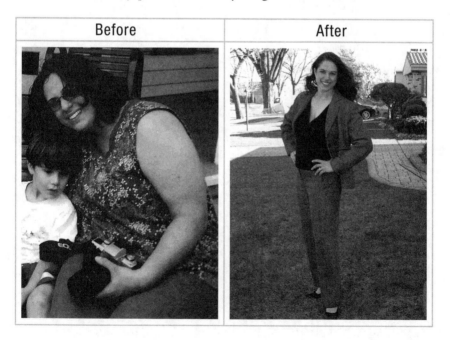

Before	After

one of my dearest friends. In general, I feel unconditionally accepted and loved.

I have lost 110 pounds with First Place 4 Health and have kept it off for two years. I have learned, and I continually relearn, that in my own strength I can do nothing, especially when it comes to losing weight and keeping it off. God is faithful; He holds my hand and helps me. He has given me a hope and a future!

PART 4

Strength: Seeking Balance Physically

When you picked up this book, did you flip to this section first?

Years ago, I probably would have. If you're like me, you want to lose weight fast—so it's a natural temptation to pick up a book on weight loss and automatically skip to the section that tells you about diet, nutrition and exercise.

The goal in First Place 4 Health, however, is to live a balanced life in all areas, not just the physical.

Learning to live a balanced life is a process—and the physical component is important to that process—but so are the other parts. If you haven't read the chapters that lead up to this section, I encourage you to go back and take your time along the way.

In the next chapters, we'll show you what it means to live a balanced life physically.

Chapter 9

Healthy Eating

Sounds like a simple question, but have you ever stopped to consider *what* you eat and *how much* you eat?

Kay Smith, who was a longtime First Place employee, described to me her lifestyle before joining the program. Every day when Kay got off work at 2:00 P.M., she drove to a fast-food restaurant where she ordered two hamburgers fixed two different ways, along with an order of onion rings and fries (so the person taking the order wouldn't suspect that all this food was for her—as if that mattered to anybody). She would eat the food on the drive home.

Several hours later, Kay prepared dinner for her family. She had grown up in a home where everything was fried—meat, potatoes, even bread—and Kay always cooked this way for her family. As Kay fixed dinner, she always fixed extra so that she could snack along the way—in other words, as she prepared dinner, she actually ate dinner.

Then the family sat down to eat, and Kay would join them in the meal.

Then there was more snacking after dinner until bed.

Kay said of the experience, "I had absolutely no idea the quantity of food I was putting in my body every day."

When Kay joined First Place, she weighed 265 pounds. She needed to learn what to eat and how much to eat. And she knew that God not only wanted to help her lose weight but also to heal her from the inside out.

As Kay progressed in the program, she began to explore some of the reasons why she had been eating so much. Growing up, Kay was one of four daughters. The oldest daughter was the grandmother's favorite.

The youngest daughter was the mother's favorite. Neither of those girls had weight problems. But the two middle girls had weight problems. Kay was one of the middle girls.

After she began First Place, Kay actually moved back near her sisters for a while and was able to work on some of the issues that had caused feelings of insecurity during her early years.

Eventually, Kay lost 90 pounds. She has learned how to eat in a healthy way, and she knows what a balanced lifestyle is all about.

You can journey down a similar path to success. That simple question, "What do you eat and how much do you eat?" forms the foundation of what First Place 4 Health teaches about healthy eating. We want to make things as simple as possible, so what we teach about healthy eating boils down to this:

Healthy eating is all about eating the right kind of food and the right amount of food.

That's it—quality and quantity.

I realize that food consumption can be related to an intricate web of problems. If you've always had a weight problem, there's usually a good reason behind it. It could be that you never felt loved or secure as a child. Perhaps you were abused physically, emotionally, verbally or sexually. Perhaps you were hurt somewhere along the way, and food became a refuge for you. Maybe food feels like the only thing you can control in a life that's out of control. (Nobody can tell you how much or what you eat.)

That's why at First Place 4 Health we invite you to give us a year. It may take awhile to lift the lid to your inner life and discover what's going on inside. It's crucial to get at the motivation for your behavior and let the Lord transform you from the inside out. That's part of the process. Learning to live a balanced life doesn't happen overnight, but the invitation is to learn to live differently from the way you've been living.

If you've tried everything else, ask the Lord to help you. With His power, you can make the changes necessary to live a balanced life.

The First Place 4 Health Live It food plan is not about going on a diet. You can have every kind of food, and you won't get hungry choosing from the bountiful variety of God's naturally sweet fruits, crunchy and colorful vegetables, tasty whole grains, nuts and seeds, as well as low-fat dairy, lean meats, poultry and fish! And with healthy eating comes freedom. There are so many foods that can fit into a balanced lifestyle! We're going to teach you about quality and quantity—the two most important factors in learning to eat healthy.

Stay with us, and we'll show you how to truly live.

A Serious Problem

I recently watched a show on TV—I don't remember the name, but it was about women who looked back on funny mishaps during their wedding ceremonies.

Most of the women had given birth to a baby or two by the time the interviews took place. I don't even remember the incidents from the women's weddings, but what struck me most vividly was how different each woman looked now compared to her wedding picture. Every single woman had gained weight. Many had gained a lot of weight.

Why does that pattern seem so natural to us—get married, have a child or two and gain 40 pounds? Why does that harmful pattern not spur us to action instead of resignation? Have you ever considered all the complications that can arise from overeating? If you're overweight, you're more likely to develop a number of potentially serious health problems, including:

- *High blood pressure.*

- *Diabetes.* Obesity is a leading cause of type 2 Diabetes. Diabetes can cause a host of problems, including loss of eyesight, kidney failure and the need for amputation of limbs.

- *Abnormal blood fats,* which can contribute to atherosclerosis— the buildup of fatty deposits in arteries throughout your body. Atherosclerosis puts you at risk of coronary artery disease and stroke.

- *Coronary artery disease.* Excess weight causes a buildup of fatty deposits in arteries that supply blood to your heart. Over time these deposits can narrow your heart's arteries, so less blood flows to your heart. Diminished blood flow to your heart can cause chest pain (angina). Complete blockage can lead to a heart attack.

- *Stroke.* If a blood clot forms in a narrowed artery in your brain, it can block blood flow to an area of your brain. The result is a stroke. Being obese raises your risk of stroke.

- *Osteoarthritis.* This joint disorder most often affects the knees, hips and lower back. Excess weight puts extra pressure on these joints and wears away the cartilage that protects them, resulting in joint pain and stiffness.

- *Sleep Apnea.* This serious condition causes a person to stop breathing for short periods during sleep, and to snore heavily. The upper airway is blocked during sleep, which results in frequent waking at night and subsequent drowsiness during the day. Most people with sleep apnea are overweight, which contributes to a large neck and narrowed airway.

- *Cancer.* Many types of cancer are associated with being overweight. In women, these can include cancers of the breast, uterus, cervix, ovaries and gallbladder. Overweight men have a particularly higher risk of cancers of the colon, rectum and the prostate.

- *Fatty liver disease.* When you're obese, fats can build up in your liver. This fatty accumulation can lead to inflammation and scarring of the liver, which can cause cirrhosis of the liver, even if you're not a heavy alcohol drinker.

- *Gallbladder disease.* Because overweight people may produce more cholesterol, which can be deposited in the gallbladder, the risk of gallstones is higher in obese people. Fast weight loss—more than 3 pounds a week—also can increase the risk of gallstones.

Being overweight is sometimes smiled at or shrugged off as just a natural part of the aging process. But I hope you realize that being overweight is serious business. It's not just about cosmetic concerns. Obesity is life threatening. In fact, approximately 300,000 deaths each year are attributed to obesity. Being obese is not the way you were designed to be!

So what do you do if you need to lose weight?

You have to decide to change—and change for the long haul. You've got to accept where you are and be willing to make the choices necessary to begin walking on the path to healing and health.

The Live It Plan

At First Place 4 Health we don't *die*-it. We *live*-it!

The Live It Plan is the name for the nutrition and exercise component of the First Place 4 Health program. We'll talk about the exercise component in another chapter. You'll learn about the nutrition component of the plan at group meetings, but we'll talk about it a bit here as well.

The Live It nutrition plan is simple. It's something you can incorporate into your lifestyle forever. Based on credible science and common sense, it provides you with 100-percent fad-free, gimmickless advice that will not only help you lose weight but will also pave the way for better overall health.

In most weight-loss programs, a person typically has his or her own meals; everyone else in the family eats whatever they want. But with the Live It plan, your whole family can eat the same way. It's all good, healthy, tasty food. Eating the right quality and the right quantity of food can become a way of life that your whole family can enjoy.

The First Place 4 Health rule of thumb is moderation in all things. We take the rigidity out of eating to lose weight. You can have an occasional piece of cake, or two cookies, or whatever. (Just as long as eating two cookies doesn't lead you to eat the whole bag.) If it does, then you need to look at the reasons behind this kind of eating. Most likely there is something out of balance in the emotional quadrant of life, and you can get to the root of the problem by lifting the lid of your inner life, as we talked about earlier. The point is that eating the Live It way is about developing an individual, healthy-eating food plan that you can live with for the rest of your life.

The time for lasting change is now. If you've spent your life eating as you hover over your sink, or gulping fast food in your car, we want to help you change that.

The following list is what we call "The First Place 4 Health Nutrition Top 10." These are suggestions to help you begin to think in a new way about what is healthy eating. You don't have to memorize this list—we'll walk you through various parts of each guideline at your weekly First Place 4 Health meetings.

The First Place 4 Health Nutrition Top 10

1. Set Realistic, Individual Goals

Losing 50 pounds before a reunion that's three weeks away is not a realistic goal. At First Place 4 Health, we encourage you to take an honest look at where you are now and where you desire to be in the future. Embrace the reality that your weight-loss journey may last much longer than 12 weeks. Set your goals accordingly and remember that gradual weight loss is the most effective kind (no more than 2 pounds per week).

Don't focus only on the scale. There are many other indicators of health besides your weight. Are you becoming stronger? Do you have more energy throughout the day? Have you seen any change in your cholesterol level or blood pressure?

Health and wellness are not determined solely by weight. We'll help you set true goals to live healthily for the rest of your life.

2. Plan Ahead and Prioritize

Your health can be directly related to where you live or work and who you hang around with.

For instance, if your idea of a Friday fun night with friends includes a huge meal at a favorite restaurant followed by a movie with all the fatty treats, that's going to catch up with you sooner rather than later. Your social environment is critical to making or breaking the healthy habits you're trying to develop.

In fact, the social support you have (or don't have) can be a huge factor in your success. You need to encourage others and be encouraged by others to make positive changes in your everyday life.

If you struggle with drinking soda throughout the day because there's a machine in the company break room, maybe the solution is simply to not go in the break room anymore. One way to promote healthy eating is to make nutritious items available in your physical environment. If you don't have healthy options to choose from, chances are you won't choose them at all.

You have to give your health high priority and intentionally prepare your home, your office, your car and your calendar to be a safe haven for healthy eating.

3. Concentrate on Quality

We often apply moral labels to foods. A carrot is "good." A doughnut is "bad." You feel guilty when you eat "bad" foods and vow to never eat "bad" foods again if you slip up.

But deprivation diets rarely lead to true discipline. There is a much healthier way to think about food. Instead of bad and good, consider foods in terms of their quality ("unhealthy," "healthy" or "healthiest") and how often you should eat them ("rarely," "sometimes," "often").

This method eliminates the notion that certain foods must be cut out completely. Broccoli, for example, would fall into the "healthiest" and "often" categories. Cheese would fall into the "healthy" and "sometimes" categories. Doughnuts would fall into the "unhealthy" and "rarely" categories (but could still have a place in every healthy diet—but not a prominent place!).

Thinking of and labeling foods without moral implications also teaches us to play a conscious role in our eating habits. God gives us a mind to discern, and we have more than enough knowledge about what is healthy and what is not—we just have to apply this knowledge.

4. Quantity Counts

When you join a First Place 4 Health group, the first two weeks will be spent discussing food and healthy eating. Many of us suffer from portion distortion, especially in regard to unhealthy foods. We will show you what an appropriate portion size is by reading labels, measuring portions at first and making educated estimates.

We'll also give you tips for dining out, such as cutting your portions in half at most restaurants or splitting them with a friend or family member. Forget super-sizing anything. It's too expensive to your waistline.

We'll show you how to lower your fat and sugar intake. We teach portion control and give you guidelines for that. We will also give you hints about food preparation that make the First Place 4 Health program easy to use.

Our goal at First Place 4 Health is never to put you on some sort of restrictive, low-calorie diet that emphasizes eating celery all day and feeling miserable all the time. Nobody can live like that, and besides, a celery-only diet wouldn't be healthy. God has given us many wonderful foods to explore and eat. At First Place 4 Health, we include all the food groups in their proper amounts. We're going to teach you how to eat.

5. Begin with a Healthy Breakfast

Many people skip breakfast; but even when you're not hungry, it's important to jump-start your metabolism for the day with a balanced breakfast.

People who eat breakfast generally burn 4 to 6 percent more calories than those who don't. Not only does eating a healthy breakfast help your body to work more efficiently, but it also protects you from overeating during the rest of the day.

6. Choose Better Beverages

Your beverage choice impacts your weight and your health. Most Americans only count the calories they get from solid foods; but did you know that beverages supply nearly a quarter of our total calories?

Sadly, the largest contributors of these calories are nutrient-poor sweetened beverages, according to national surveys.

We'll show you how to replace beverages such as regular soda, pre-sweetened teas, and fruit-flavored drinks with nutritious ones with fewer calories per serving: low-fat milk, 100-percent juice with no added sugar, and that wonderful beverage—water!

7. Spread Your Calories Around

We'll show you how to develop an estimated daily calorie level. Once you have this estimate, you can take your estimate and divide it by 3 meals and 2 snacks. They don't have to be equal in calories, but the goal is to eat every 4 to 6 hours when awake rather than waiting until you're stomach is growling uncontrollably. (You may need to eat every 2 to 3 hours if you deal with blood sugar control.)

8. Balance Your Plate

You'll learn how to divide your meals and snacks into three categories. Include some *quality* carbohydrate, protein and fat at every meal in the appropriate *quantities*. Balancing your plate will create a more nutritionally balanced and complete meal or snack.

9. Read Food Labels

We'll teach you to become a proactive, health-conscious consumer by reading and comparing food labels, nutrition facts and ingredients lists. Few of us take advantage of the buying power available to us every day. Nutrition facts are provided at most restaurants and even online. Everything you need to know to make an informed decision about any food, from applesauce to zucchini bread, can be found by simply flipping the item over and reading the label (including the ingredients).

10. Practice Mindfulness

When you keep a written record of what you eat and drink, and why, you make yourself aware of your motivations and choices. Are you eating because you're truly hungry or because you're tired, bored or upset? By following the Live It plan, you'll learn to eat slowly and savor your meals. You'll relearn what hunger really feels like and listen to your internal hunger cues—and stop when you are full. God designed your body with thousands of fascinating intricacies that all have a purpose. Trust your gut—God made that, too!

Our busy lifestyle has led us to rely on fast foods and frozen dinners. Fat content is high in many of these and, unfortunately, even the healthiest frozen dinners are usually high in sodium. If you plan ahead, home-cooked meals can be prepared just as quickly and at a much lower cost.

Other weight-loss plans provide food with proper nutrition, but you have to buy the food from the plan distributors. These plans work for a period of time because they provide the right amount of food. But they don't teach you to make choices. Most people don't want to eat prepared foods indefinitely. In every one of these plans, a time comes when you have to begin to eat for yourself, but you haven't been prepared to do it. Also, these plans can be expensive and lack variety. With any of these systems, if you begin to make your own choices again but have not changed your old patterns or mindset, it will be all too easy to revert to old patterns of eating.

First Place 4 Health uses the USDA MyPyramid food guidance system. Proper food selection in the right quantity is the key to keeping your body strong and healthy. We'll show you what that means.

Your Plan Today

As you learn to examine the quality and quantity of the foods you eat, you will never want to return to your old habits. When you follow the Live It plan, you are in for a treat, not a trial. God created us for success.

He created us for victory. By trusting in Christ and choosing to make beneficial choices every day, you are going to have the strength to win.

You can make the changes necessary to start on this journey today. By choosing the positive direction in front of you right now, you can start to get your life on track physically. The pounds will come off and they will stay off. Better yet, your life will manifest balance, and you will have the skills to live the amazing life you were created to live.

Checklist for Success

• Start using a daily record of your food consumption. You will be amazed at how this tool will help you make better choices in what you eat and how much you eat.

• Take extra pounds seriously! Obesity can lead to a host of complications that can even threaten your life.

• Healthy eating is all about eating the right quality and quantity of food.

Chapter 10

Just Move

A woman in her early 60s had been coming to First Place 4 Health for three years and was seeing minimal success. All she could ever seem to lose was 5 pounds, and then she'd gain it right back as soon as each 12-week session was over. She knew what the solution was—we all did. It was just a matter of her doing it.

"I'm just plain ol' lazy," this woman told Vicki Heath, our First Place Networking Coordinator, when Vicki asked her why she never exercised. You have to appreciate this woman's honesty—there are a million excuses people give for not exercising. At least she owned up to hers.

Vicki and the woman began praying about her lack of exercise. The woman started walking for 20 minutes, four times per week on a treadmill she had in her basement.

And in 12 weeks she lost 12 pounds!

That was all the difference she needed—just a little bit of exercise. I'm so proud of this woman. Notice that she didn't begin training to run a marathon right away or lift huge amounts of weight. All she did was walk moderately on a treadmill, on a regular basis.

That was all it took. Small steps count up to big rewards.

Unenthusiastic Exercisers

I'm convinced that it's impossible to live a balanced life unless you exercise. The body was designed to move. Your call to exercise is one of the most significant invitations you'll ever receive to bring balance to your life. Yet it can also be one of the most challenging.

You may hate the very thought of exercise. You may have never exercised a day in your life. *Exercise is only for jocks*, you've always told yourself.

Maybe you used to exercise a long time ago, but the thought of exercising now terrifies you, or overwhelms you, or just makes you want to go lie down.

Maybe you love to exercise, but you've convinced yourself that you are too busy—you just can't cram anything more into your day.

Maybe you have some physical disabilities that make exercise a challenge. You'd love to have the strong body you once had, but most movement today is painful. What do you do then?

Vicki Heath is also a certified fitness trainer and has led group fitness classes for more than a decade. She has kept a list of reasons people have given her over the years for why they don't want to exercise. Beyond the obvious excuses such as "It's too hot (or cold)" or "I'm too tired (or busy)," her list includes:

- I need to do laundry.
- My dog is sick.
- I don't have any shoes.
- I don't have any money.
- I have to cook supper for my husband.
- I need to get my nails done.
- My fat jiggles when I run.
- It shoots my morning.
- It shoots my evening.
- I'll miss my favorite TV program.

I've come up with some excuses myself over the years. My problem is that I hate to sweat; my hair gets wet and I have to wash it. I've learned to ignore my excuses and exercise anyway. Exercise has become as daily to me as brushing my teeth or going to work. I can promise you that my day is always better when I choose to exercise than when I choose not to.

What helps keep me motivated is that I love the way I *feel* because I exercise. I love the *results*. I love keeping my weight in check and having more energy throughout the day. I love how exercise clears my mind and relieves stress and tension. I love not losing muscle mass, bone density or flexibility.

And *exercise* works! Exercise helps you live the life you truly want to live. I've experienced this firsthand. The women in my family have a long history of osteoarthritis, a disease that is spurred forward when a person doesn't exercise. My mother had the disease and was in a wheelchair the last three years of her life. My sister, seven years older than me, died when she was only 60. She had osteoarthritis in all of her joints, including her fingers, elbows and knees—it was very painful for her. My maternal grandmother had osteoarthritis in her spine and was in a wheelchair the last six years of her life.

During my last checkup, the doctor said I was in top shape. At 65, I have just a trace of the disease in my back and neck, but nothing major. I can move freely. I'm not in pain. I can walk up and down stairs and sit for two hours in a car each day without my back bothering me. I can bend over without effort to pick up my great-grandchild to give him a cuddle. Most important, I can continue to do the work God has called me to do. I've been exercising regularly for the past 20 years, and I credit much of my good health now to that fact.

Why Exercise Is Such a Good Thing

You might not have a family history of osteoarthritis, but everybody has personal reasons why regular exercise simply makes a lot of sense.

A 52-year-old man who recently joined First Place 4 Health described his reason as simply "wanting to not miss out." His whole life had revolved around *not* moving. He would get up in the morning and drive to work where he took the elevator to his office and sat all day. He'd drive home at day's end and sit down for the rest of the evening until bedtime. His lifestyle wasn't far from being totally sedentary.

The problem came to a head the day his son graduated from college. To get to the auditorium where the ceremonies were held, the man had to walk across a parking lot. Parking was tight that day and the man had to park near the back of the lot—about a quarter mile's walk from the entrance.

The man couldn't do it. He couldn't walk that distance. "It was incredibly humiliating," he said. He had to rest while a family member went back, got the car, drove him to the entrance, let him out, then went back and re-parked the car.

That was the catalyst for this man to get moving. He signed up for a general movement class at a fitness center. He started to do a bit of kickboxing. At first he couldn't even lift two 5-pound weights in each hand over his head. But in just six weeks, he was lifting 8 pounds above his head for 10 repetitions. He also improved his range of motion. His balance and coordination increased. And he could walk for more than 10 minutes without needing to stop and rest.

That's success!

The benefits of exercise are so far-reaching. Take a minute to go through the checklist below. Tick off any and all areas that you can relate to.

I want to lose weight. ☐ Yes ☐ No
It's virtually impossible to lose weight without exercising. Even simple movements are beneficial.

I care about my heart. ☐ Yes ☐ No

Statistics show that heart disease kills 750,000 people in America annually. Even a moderate amount of exercise helps your heart.

I care about having strong bones. ☐ Yes ☐ No

Exercise, together with a healthy calcium intake, has been shown to prevent osteoporosis. Weight-bearing exercise, like running, walking and weight lifting are particularly important.

I don't want clogged arteries. ☐ Yes ☐ No

Exercise reduces LDL cholesterol, the kind that clogs arteries.

I'm concerned about my blood pressure. ☐ Yes ☐ No

Exercise lowers high blood pressure.

I need to reduce my stress. ☐ Yes ☐ No

Exercise is an excellent de-stressor.

I hate getting sick. ☐ Yes ☐ No

Exercise helps prevents colds and reduces the duration of a cold. Thirty minutes of brisk walking each day is enough to reap the benefits of a boosted immune system. Exercise also helps asthma sufferers, diabetics, headache sufferers, and reduces the risk of getting cancer.

I want to live as well as I can no matter my age. ☐ Yes ☐ No

Exercise has anti-aging effects. It enhances blood flow to the brain, keeps reaction times quicker and improves coordination. Exercise improves reasoning and memory. It improves lung function. It reduces the risk of chronic lifestyle diseases and helps prevent stroke.

I want a better sex life. ☐ Yes ☐ No

Medical research indicates that the fitter you are, the better your sex life is. The reasons seem to be twofold: (1) Psychologically you feel better about yourself and are more inclined toward sex, and (2) being physically fit improves libido, blood circulation and sexual functioning.

I want to sleep better. ☐ Yes ☐ No
Exercise improves sleep patterns and reduces insomnia.

I want to look better. ☐ Yes ☐ No
Exercise can improve your physique, posture, muscle tone and more.

I just want to feel better. ☐ Yes ☐ No
Exercise can lift your mood, counter depression, clear your mind and sort out your thoughts, and improve your self-esteem. You simply feel better the more you move.

How about you? Take a moment to examine your life. In the space below, write down the excuses you are prone to give for not exercising, and then list your top three reasons for wanting to exercise.

The reason I often don't exercise is because . . .

_____

_____

_____

My top three reasons for needing to exercise are . . .
1. _____
2. _____
3. _____

Congratulations. Honesty about yourself is a key step in the process of creating a balanced life. Knowing what you're up against and what motivates you are key pieces of the journey.

Your Exercise Invitation

When we talk about exercise, we're really talking about three components. Each one is an important part of the process. The three components are strength training, flexibility training and cardiovascular training.

Training for Strength

When people hear the words "strength training," they sometimes envision a muscle-bound body-builder pumping heavy iron. But really, training for strength is something everybody is invited to do, regardless of his or her level of physical fitness. You don't have to buy barbells; two cans of vegetables from the pantry will do!

When you train for strength, you put an overload on your muscles and bones that causes the muscle to become stronger and the bone to become more durable.

Normal everyday activity seldom puts an overload on your muscles or bones. So training for strength requires intentional targeting of each of your major muscle groups, such as your back and abdominals.

Training for strength also increases your endurance—something everybody can use more of. Imagine all the practical things you could do if you had more endurance—play with a child or grandchild longer, sit at an office job without fatigue, stand in line at a grocery store and have your legs not hurt.

Although I don't hear this from the men, women tell me they don't want to train for strength because they don't want big muscles—they're trying to get smaller, not larger. The truth is that working with heavier weights can create larger muscles, but working with smaller weights doing more repetitions can actually create more compact muscles. It helps trim and tighten you. Lean muscle tissue takes up less space than fat.

Training for strength also increases your body's metabolism so that you burn more calories when your body is at rest. Fat is inert—it just sits there taking up space—but muscle needs fuel to burn.

Exercise physiologist and author Dr. Richard Couey has done studies on women who have done years of yo-yo dieting. Their metabolism
was so low that they were stuck and couldn't seem to lose any weight.
Dr. Couey discovered that if these women broke their exercise into two
or three sessions a day, it jump-started their metabolism. For instance,
if you normally walk for one hour, walk 20 minutes morning, noon and
night. This arrangement also works when you've lost weight but hit
a plateau.

Flexibility Training

Flexibility refers to lengthening the connective tissues in your body,
which will allow greater freedom of movement.

Why might you want greater freedom of movement? There are all
the obvious reasons—like ease of reaching into the back seat of your car
to pick something up. Flexibility also reduces the risk of injury and
reduces muscle tension and soreness.

Have you ever thought of the physical and mental relaxation that
can come from greater flexibility? So many of us are living at warp
speed in a terrible body. If we would just take the time to slow down,
breathe and stretch, the effects would be amazing.

Part of being flexible is linked to gender and genetics; for instance,
some people have longer hamstrings than others. Women tend to be
more flexible than men, particularly in the hip joints. Regardless of
genetics or gender, flexibility is about starting where you are. Anyone
can learn to be more flexible. And anyone can take just five minutes a
day to stretch.

Cardiovascular Training

Cardiovascular training is aerobic exercise for your heart and circulation. It increases and strengthens the amount of blood your heart

pumps through your body, bringing it more oxygen. If your heart is weak, it has to pump more times to get enough oxygen to the body. That's why a professional athlete's resting pulse rate is normally very low—his or her heart is so strong that it pumps enormous amounts of blood through the body every time it beats. Aerobic exercise includes activities like walking, jogging, swimming and bicycling but can be any exercise that elevates your heart rate to a training level and keeps it there for 20 minutes. (Training heart rate is calculated based on a percentage of your maximum heart rate, which is determined by subtracting your age from 220.)

A good target goal is to exercise aerobically three to five times a week while also incorporating flexibility and strength training into your lifestyle.

We also recommend a walking program called "10,000 Steps to Wellness." Walking is so easy—it comes naturally, it's inexpensive, it can be done anywhere and it doesn't require practice or special equipment.

With the 10,000 steps program, you can measure your progress by wearing a pedometer, which traces your steps by detecting body motion; even small steps can speed you toward your fitness goals. Ten thousand steps equal approximately five miles, so build up to the goal gradually. To begin, establish a baseline of steps by measuring the number of steps you take in an average day. Record the findings for three days; add them up and divide by three. This will be your baseline standard. Increase your steps gradually by adding to your baseline average—approximately 200 to 1,000 steps a day.

A young mom who comes to a First Place 4 Health class has two kids: a 3-year-old and an 18-month-old. Her husband is in the military and is often gone, so her goal is simply to keep up with her kids—to not get worn out—while her husband is away. She's found that the pedometer is a good way of keeping track of her exercise. Playing at the playground with her kids for half an hour is more intensive than a 30-minute walk!

Exercise doesn't have to be programmed; it can be a daily part of an active life. All activity is cumulative!

Here are suggestions for getting more aerobic exercise:

- Park at the back of a parking lot. There are always good spots open, and you'll get in lots of steps on the way into and out of the store.
- Whenever you can, use stairs instead of an elevator or escalator.
- Stop using the remote and get up to change the channel on your TV.
- If you've got a layover on a flight, don't just sit down and wait—use that time to walk around the airport.

Look for ways to incorporate movement into every area of your life. Be creative. Small steps add up.

Let's Get Practical

What can you do today to motivate yourself toward success in this area? Let me suggest a few tips.

Set goals for yourself. Setting a goal helps keep you on target. Goals are always personal and usually have a time limit built in. A goal could be to run a 5K race in a year's time, or maybe to walk around the block by the time a month has come and gone.

A First Place 4 Health group on the East Coast set up a fun program awhile back called "Walk to Bethlehem." The program was held during the months leading up to Christmas. The idea was for several First Place 4 Health groups to band together and keep track of how many miles each person walked each day. The miles would be tallied with the goal of walking 5,100 miles—roughly the distance from the East Coast of America to Bethlehem. Each person kept an exercise log. And they did it! They did the mileage.

Focus on the results of exercise. If you find exercise difficult, keep in mind the big picture of why you're exercising. Focus on the positive results of what exercise will do for you. Picture in your mind how you feel when you step on the scale and see that you've lost another 5 pounds. Or envision what it's like to fit into that smaller size of jeans.

Stop thinking of exercise as a punishment. Some people think things such as, *Well, I've just pigged out on cheesecake; I need to go run around the block.*

This seldom works well. Whenever you view exercise as a punishment or even a purging of excess, it casts a negative shadow on the whole process. Exercise works best when it's viewed as a regular, positive part of life.

Avoid the "toos." That means avoid too much, too soon, too fast. The *toos* are a recipe for disaster.

Invest in a good pair of exercise shoes. A good pair of shoes is perhaps the most important piece of exercise equipment you'll need. Cost is not an indicator of whether a shoe is right for you. The critical factor is locating a shoe that fits: one that is not too wide, too short or too long. Serious exercisers do not look like they've just stepped out of a fashion catalog; usually they look pretty grubby—but they're comfortable.

From my perspective you don't need to spend a lot of money to exercise. Although it is possible to spend as much on your exercise clothes and shoes as the rest of your wardrobe, all you really need are some loose fitting pants, a shirt and a pair of comfortable, stable shoes.

Keep an exercise log. I keep a personal log of when and how much I exercise. It works for me. If I miss a week, I just write across that page what was going on and why I couldn't exercise. At the end of the year, my goal is to never exercise less than I did the year before. That way I'm always working to increase my fitness.

Pick a time that's right for you. When you're doing programmed exercise, pick a time that works for your schedule. Although my best time to exercise is in the morning, because it fits better with my work day, if you have young children, the morning might be the worst possible time to exercise. You will need to experiment and find the time of day that works best for you. The main thing is to choose a time that you can stick with on a regular basis.

Some young parents use their children as an excuse not to exercise. Yet children love to go out and walk and ride bikes. There's no better family time than when the entire family exercises together. It thrills me to see families exercising together. Not only are the parents doing something that will increase their own health and well-being, but their children are also learning a lifetime habit of healthy choices.

If you don't have children, there are other benefits for you. Husbands and wives have told me they never had time to truly communicate with each other until they began exercising together.

Exercise is good for you at any age and at any time. The main thing is to pick a time when you can be faithful to exercise. If you can exercise regularly after work, then that's the time for you. Some studies have revealed that if you work out in the late afternoon, you will be less hungry at dinner.

Your Plan for Today

Recently, we had a 70-year-old join a First Place 4 Health group. She was about 100 pounds overweight. Both of her knees had been surgically replaced and she had a great deal of difficulty getting around. She knew that she needed to exercise, but it was her biggest challenge in living a balanced life.

The woman lived on a little island about a half mile from the beach. Her first goal was to walk to the beach and back—an entire mile. She hadn't walked a mile for years. She started out walking just a few steps a day. Each day she went a little farther.

In 7 months time she had lost 40 pounds and reached her exercise goal as well. I'm so proud of this woman. To me, she's a tremendous athlete, someone who demonstrates true effort and embodies a champion spirit. Just think of how much more difficult it is for her to walk than for an able-bodied person. In the end, she accomplished her goal by taking one step at a time.

The time to get physically fit is now. It doesn't matter where you are; start with what you can do. Just start moving. Begin by walking a short distance every day. Swim. Bike. Play golf. Or just walk more than you do today.

You can do it.

When you exercise on a regular basis, it changes your life. Your invitation is to put on your shoes right now and walk out your front door.

Checklist for Success

- Weight loss is a physical issue definitely, but it's not solely a physical issue. The goal is living a balanced life—spiritually, mentally, emotionally and physically.

- Giving an excuse for why not to exercise is taking the easy way out. The benefits of exercise are so enormous that you can't ignore them.

- Exercise involves three parts: strength training, flexibility, and cardiovascular fitness. A good exercise routine involves all three.

- Exercise is cumulative. Start small and start today.

Chapter 11

I've Changed My Mind

Once upon a time, a married couple decided to lose weight. We'll call them Bernice and Bartholomew. This is what they did:

When January 1 came around, Bernice and Bartholomew made New Year's resolutions to shed those extra pounds, just like every year.

First, they looked for the newest fad diet and signed up. Step 1 was to drastically reduce their calorie intake. So they opened their cupboards and threw everything away, just as the diet program instructed them to do. Most of the food in there—the food that they liked to eat and were used to eating—was labeled "bad" food. It was tempting to eat, and tasty, but off-limits, according to the diet program.

The diet program told them they should only eat "good" foods, so Bernice and Bartholomew raced to sign up for their supply of pre-processed, pre-packaged weight-loss foods ordered from the diet company. The company promised quick results if you ate only their food, and that's exactly what Bernice and Bartholomew were looking for. Speed. It seemed like a no-brainer.

Next, they knew they needed to exercise, so they decided to set their alarm clocks for three hours earlier than they usually got up in the morning. The following morning, Bernice and Bartholomew donned new workout suits and headed out for a 10-mile jog. They weren't runners by nature, but running was the only exercise that came to mind. The new exercise felt agonizing—too much, too soon—but they had always heard the adage "No pain, no gain," so they pressed on.

That same morning, hours later, they arrived back at their house, sweaty, exhausted, footsore and absolutely miserable. They looked unhappy and felt unhappy, and that's how they decided to spend the rest of their day. They knew they could only be happy if they were thin. Everybody knows that—right?

Bernice and Bartholomew seldom talked to each other during the course of their diet, let alone talk to anyone else about it. They believed that weight loss is something you do alone. It certainly wasn't something to do within a group of other people.

Bernice and Bartholomew set no goals for themselves other than to lose weight. They gave no thought to what their lifestyle would look like after they lost the weight. Their only hope was to persevere long enough at the diet in order to lose the weight they needed to lose.

Although Bernice and Bartholomew were Christians, they never prayed about their diet or their health. Surely God had bigger concerns. Besides—eating a lot was a regular part of many of their church functions. Potlucks were all about piling your plate as high as you could. Sugary doughnuts and caffeine-laden coffee were a part of every Sunday School hour. Just look at their pastor. He was extremely overweight and the godliest person they knew. Surely he couldn't be that far off track.

As the diet continued, temptations continued to come across Bernice and Bartholomew's path. Their diet was difficult, but they had faith that if they just gritted their teeth hard enough, they would persevere. So that's what they did—buckled down and tried harder. Boy, that diet was hard! Temptations were everywhere. But they knew that if they just had enough willpower, they would succeed.

Down deep, they knew there must be some reason they had a continual battle with weight gain, and they felt nothing but guilt about all their horrible habits. They must be badly flawed people. Exercise was a punishment, but they continued quoting the "No pain, no gain" maxim to each other and staggered on.

All in all, their diet felt too strict and confining, but they knew it was going to work because that's what diets always felt like.

Bernice and Bartholomew followed their diet for exactly two weeks. By mid-January, they had dropped five pounds and were ecstatic, so they went out to celebrate at an all-you-can-eat buffet. Diet over! There was much rejoicing. Everything returned to "normal."

Two weeks later, they had regained the five pounds lost and put on two additional pounds. Bartholomew and Bernice knew they needed to do something again. So they went searching for another diet.

And so it continued for many years . . .

Winds of Change

If the story of Bernice and Bartholomew had been at the front of this book, and you hadn't yet read any of the First Place 4 Health philosophy on how to live a balanced life, maybe their story wouldn't appear all that strange to you. But already, you've begun to see health in a new light.

I'm not suggesting that First Place 4 Health has an exclusive corner on a new way of thinking. Fortunately, the winds of change are blowing through a new generation of researchers, physicians and health-promotion specialists who are diligently working to change our thinking by promoting what they call the new weight paradigm.

We at First Place 4 Health welcome this new thinking. God is all about change, whenever change is for the better. He is ever working in our minds and hearts to transform us to a new way of thinking by the power of His Word and influence of His Holy Spirit. The new weight paradigm invites us to change our minds about several long-held ways of thinking.

I hope you've seen new ways of thinking all through this book, but let me suggest a couple of thoughts that summarize the forefront of the new weight paradigm.

Change Your Mind About "Thin"

At the foundation of this new approach to weight loss is a change in assumptions about what it means to be healthy.

For most of the twentieth century, people assumed that thinness was essential for both good health and happiness. "You can't be too thin" is an expression you've probably heard before (or some variation of it).

If "you can't be too thin" is the truth, then the assumption is that those who are not thin must lack willpower and either eat too much or not exercise enough. Therefore, the solution to being overweight is to simply eat less and exercise more.

It sounds good on the surface, but as we are finding, and as statistics bear out, it's not that simple.

We do know that diets rarely work. Those who have tried them—and failed—know this, and now physicians and weight researchers are acknowledging it as well. Factors such as genetics and physiological mechanisms are finally receiving due credit for their roles in determining body shape and size and a body's ability to shed extra pounds.

If you're one of those people who do not lose weight quickly or who take longer to find success in your weight-loss goals, take heart. The new goal is not *thin;* the new goal is *healthy.* And *healthy* can look a lot of different ways.

Healthy does not mean being obese or overweight, but it's probably not stick-skinny either, unless you're a stick-skinny person by nature. There can be a lot of factors that determine what *healthy* looks like for you.

Change Your Mind About Healthy

We've just said that the new goal is *healthy,* but did you know that the understanding of what it means to be *healthy* is also changing?

The new weight paradigm focuses on things other than weight loss: healthy eating, regular exercise and an esteem and understanding of yourself that's rooted in truth: that a good God loves you and has a plan and purpose for your life.

Being healthy has less to do with a number on a scale than the ability to balance and nurture all aspects of one's life: the emotional, the mental and the spiritual, as well as the physical.

Here are three examples of the new "healthy" at work:

- *Old way of thinking:* Drastic reduction in calories is the best way to lose weight.

- *New way of thinking:* Healthy, relaxed eating in response to hunger and satiety cues is the key to developing a comfortable relationship with food and avoiding eating disorders.

- *Old way of thinking:* Exercise is punishment for my imperfect body.

- *New way of thinking:* Exercise is an excellent way to improve my health and enhance my quality of life.

- *Old way of thinking:* People need to be thin in order to be healthy and happy.

- *New way of thinking:* People naturally have different body shapes and sizes, and need to accept and be grateful for the way they were fearfully and wonderfully made by our Creator.

Change Your Mind About Accountability

In the old weight paradigm, weight loss was either something you had to do all alone without any help, or something you had to very rigidly subscribe to. Sometimes it was both of those things. Accountability was either nonexistent or fairly tight—you either made the grade or you didn't.

We've always promoted a group approach to health at First Place 4 Health, so we've been on track with that part of the new way of thinking about accountability. But we've come to believe that we've promoted the aspect of commitments perhaps too strongly in the past. We used to structure our program around nine commitments, with the goal of keeping all of them—all the time. We've eased up on that.

Don't misunderstand; commitments are not wrong. On one hand, you have to be very serious about your weight loss, which takes dedication and effort and willpower and perseverance. You can't just sit back and be complacent about your health.

At the same time, at First Place 4 Health the emphasis is never about gritting your teeth and trying harder. We want to promote a way of health that is grace-filled and peacefully successful. Health is not about punishing yourself for eating a cookie now and then, or a rigid system of dos and don'ts.

So we've begun to use the word "invitation" more and more, instead of the word "commitment." The idea is that God *invites* you to a new way of thinking about your life. He won't whack you with a brick if you eat an occasional piece of cheesecake or don't exercise one morning or don't read your Bible for one day. Christ calls us to a place of devotion to Him. His way is a lifestyle, and that lifestyle is abundant. It doesn't mean the journey will always be easy, but it does mean the journey is grace-filled. I hope you've seen that new attitude expressed all through this book.

A Closer Look at Accountability

Accountability is one of the key invitations in First Place 4 Health—that call to go the road together. Let's take a closer look at accountability and what it might look like in your life under this new way of thinking.

There's an amazing story in 1 Kings about the prophet Elijah, who stumbles at this very point.

Elijah was a blood and thunder prophet. After a whirlwind season of raising the dead, slaughtering false prophets and running up and down Mt. Carmel a few times, Elijah finally received a death threat from evil Queen Jezebel and ran for his life. So Elijah journeyed for a day into the desert where he finally collapsed from exhaustion, both from all the good he had done and also the danger he was then in.

Weakened, spent, tired and troubled, He found himself sitting under a broom tree, praying desperate prayers to God. Elijah's prayer is the prayer of a man who believed he was all alone. First Kings 19:10 records his words: "I have been very zealous for the LORD God Almighty . . . [and now] . . . I am the only one left."

It is at this point that God spoke, but probably not how Elijah would imagine. First came a powerful windstorm, but God was not in the wind. Then there was an earthquake, but God was not there either. After the earthquake came a fire, but still no sign of God. After the fire came a gentle whisper. When Elijah heard this, he pulled his cloak about him, stood at the mouth of the cave and prepared to listen to what God had to say to him.

From within the gentle whisper, God's voice gave Elijah some specific instructions about where he should go and what he should do. One of God's main communications was a gentle rebuke to Elijah that reminded him that he was not alone. God had 7,000 prophets specifically following His call at that very moment. Elijah was not alone at all.

Just like Elijah, that truth—*you are not alone*—is so very key to your own success. In First Place 4 Health, you have the opportunity to join a group of trusted friends who will help you along the journey and help hold you accountable.

Sometimes when people think of the word "accountability," they envision a pupil reporting to a strict teacher every week. In that scenario the emphasis is discipline and punishment for falling out of line.

In truth, accountability is about journeying the road together. None of us are perfect. All of us can use the encouragement that comes from interaction with other people. The concept of accountability is found all throughout Scripture.

Ecclesiastes 4:9-12 says:

Two are better than one,
Because they have a good return for their work:
If one falls down, his friend can help him up.
But pity the man who falls and has no one to help him up!
Also, if two lie down together, they will keep warm.
But how can one keep warm alone?
Through one may be overpowered, two can defend themselves.
A cord of three strands is not quickly broken.

All through the New Testament, we find examples of this as well. John 13:34 encourages us to love one another. Romans 1:12 notes how we are mutually encouraged by each other's faith. Ephesians 5:30 talks about how we are all members of Christ's Body. First Thessalonians 5:11 exhorts us to encourage each other and build each other up.

The call is clear: Journey toward health with other people. Become healthy within a community of trusted friends. First Place 4 Health offers that opportunity.

Accountability means that we walk the journey toward health together. For instance, every morning I am accountable to my good friend Becky. We have a standing date to meet in the weight room at the church, walk on the treadmill and say our verses together. There is no tension in this meeting. Becky is not grading me on my verses, nor will she punish me if I don't show up, and vice versa. We have a friendship, and our accountability is based on encouragement and walking the road together.

Also within the concept of accountability is the idea of safeguarding your life. For instance, I know a woman who loves potato chips. Whenever she buys a bag, she only eats some of the bag and throws the rest away. She knows that if the partially eaten bag is left in the house, she will be much more prone to eat the entire bag the same day. That's safeguarding—taking whatever steps are necessary to ensure your health.

Tossing a half-eaten bag of chips away might sound drastic to you if you've grown up in a generation that never threw away food. You might ask why she simply doesn't save the rest for later. Well, this woman knows that her resistance level in this area is still low, and this is part of the system she's developed to hold herself accountable.

Accountability still asks for our responsibility, yet it acknowledges that sometimes willpower alone is not enough to do the job.

I safeguard my life in various ways, both on a personal level and as a First Place 4 Health leader. For instance, one of the best ways I know to keep myself reading Scripture on a daily basis is to regularly lead a Bible study. That's what works for me. I know that each week when I face my group, I need to come prepared—and that means I've spent time with the Lord myself. Leading a Bible study is part of my accountability system. It's part of the way I lead a balanced life.

The Live It Tracker

I mentioned that we're not using the word "commitments" as much at First Place 4 Heath. The idea of "committing" to something is a positive thing as long as you know that you have flexibility within that system. But to carry through the theme that what we *learn* we then need to *live,* we changed the name of our tool for tracking daily choices from "Commitment Record" to "Live It Tracker." We've used this kind of tool for years, and it's a good one. It will help you stay on course in your health journey.

Years ago, we developed this tracking tool based on Proverbs 16:3:

Commit to the LORD whatever you do, and your plans will succeed.

That's the same spirit in which we talk about the Live It Tracker today. When your life is devoted to the Lord, your daily choices will reflect that priority.

As a participant in First Place 4 Health, every day you're invited to fill out a day's worth of the Live It Tracker. We keep these pull-out pages at the back of our Bible studies.

Essentially, a Live It Tracker is a food diary plus a record of your physical activity. On the Live It Tracker, you're invited to record the quality and quantity of what you eat and the type and length of physical activity you've done.

This record is really for your benefit, nothing more. It allows you to record your successes and difficulties each week. For instance, in the area of food, the record shows which food groups you might be lacking in, and in what areas you might be overeating.

The Live It Tracker is not about passing or failing. It's just a record of keeping track of your progress.

When I became a First Place 4 Health group leader, I didn't fill out my Live It Tracker each day. At the leaders' meetings on Wednesday nights, I would try to reconstruct my food consumption over the previous week. During one of these meetings, my leader, Dotty Brewer, said, "It's kind of hard to reconstruct a whole week in five minutes, isn't it, Carole?"

That was the reminder I needed to keep track every day. Even today, after many years of practicing the precepts of First Place 4 Health, I find it helpful to keep a Live It Tracker so that I stay on the Live It plan.

At your weekly group meeting, you will give your Live It Tracker to your leader. It's not about evaluation; it's about encouragement and consultation. The Live It Tracker becomes a method of communication between you and your leader. It's not handed over so that your leader can judge or criticize you, but so that she or he can encourage you to make good choices. One of our leaders refers to the Live It Tracker as her best friend. This record reveals trends that make a difference in her health goals.

Many people keep their Live It Tracker in their Bible study book. Others find that keeping it in their purse or organizer—or even posted on the refrigerator—is more convenient. Think of your Live It Tracker as your good friend, not a policeman. Accountability keeps us on track.

A Happier Ending

Imagine with me another scenario—one like the story at the beginning of this chapter, but this one's based on the new paradigm of healthy thinking. Once upon a time, another couple decided to lose weight. We'll call them Celeste and Chris. This is what they did:

January 1 came around, and the same as every year, Celeste and Chris used that date as a catalyst to begin a different way of doing things. They could have used any date to begin making a change, or no particular date at all. They could have simply made a decision that "today" was the day to change. A friend brought them to a First Place 4 Health program, and they signed up.

They soon discovered that losing weight is not simply about changing the numbers they saw on a scale. Celeste and Chris were surprised to learn that First Place 4 Health isn't even a diet. It's a lifestyle change that addresses their whole being—mentally, spiritually, emotionally and physically. Once their lives were in balance, the weight issues would be addressed as well.

They soon learned a simple fact upon which everything else would hinge. That fact is that God is good, and He offered Celeste and Chris a hope-filled plan for their life and future. Their invitation was to begin on that journey toward health.

Celeste and Chris were encouraged to attend weekly First Place 4 Health meetings. Sometimes they didn't feel like going, but they made a choice to journey toward health regardless of their feelings. They didn't know the people at first, but soon they made friends and found the support, encouragement and accountability necessary to make this journey.

They learned that their journey would take time and they wouldn't lose all the weight overnight. They were encouraged to be patient with the process. The key to lasting success was to make a series of small, positive choices, day after day.

It sounded funny to them at first; Celeste and Chris were not only invited to show up at the meetings, but they were also invited to be encouragers themselves. Their weight-loss journey was not just about them—they were on a mission to health, and part of health means shedding a self-centered, cruise-ship attitude that believes "it's all about them."

Celeste and Chris had always considered themselves Christians but had never before heard that God was actually interested in their lives, much less their weight. They began to pray together about their weight—it felt like a burden began to lift off their shoulders. God was good, and God was interested in every aspect of their lives.

Celeste and Chris began to read their Bibles every day, something they had never done before. It wasn't that hard to find the time. They also began to work through a First Place 4 Health Bible study together. It took about 10 to 15 minutes per day. They found real-life answers to things they had wondered about for years. For the first time in their life, they began to memorize Scripture. That was one of the best things of all. They weren't sure if they could do it at first, but once the

Scripture was in their minds, they began to see life in a different light. Old habits that had plagued them for years were not so much an issue anymore. Once Chris and Celeste changed their thoughts by getting Scripture into their minds, they began to change how they lived.

For years, Celeste and Chris had been fairly sedentary, but now they began to make small changes to add movement to their day. They parked their car farther away from stores and enjoyed the walk inside and out. They avoided escalators and took the stairs whenever they could. Each evening when they got home, they took a brisk walk in their neighborhood. They stretched before they walked. Chris also did pushups, while Celeste lifted some barbells for strength training. Exercise became a regular part of their life.

They began to learn what it meant to eat in moderation and only when they were truly hungry. They could still eat the foods they liked, but they learned how to eat moderate portions. Their new way of eating didn't feel restrictive—it felt free.

Every so often, Celeste and Chris found themselves slipping back to old habits. For instance, when Celeste's grandfather died, there was a real temptation to eat to quell the grief. Continuing to attend the weekly First Place 4 Health meeting helped them through that rough season.

In one year's time, Celeste and Chris stood on a scale and weighed themselves. They had kept track of their progress all along by using the Live It Tracker, so their new weights didn't come as a big surprise. They lost the weight they wanted to lose and knew they had the tools to keep it off forever. Additionally, their lives were changed in ways they had never dreamed possible. They had new energy and responsiveness to whatever the Lord directed them to do.

The future looked bright, and they were well on their way.

How about you? What sort of life story are you writing right now? Is it one like the story at the beginning of this chapter, or is it more like the one at the end? Your story will be unique, but when your goal is to live a balanced life with Christ at the center, it's always a story with a good journey.

Checklist for Success

- The winds of change are blowing through a new generation of researchers, physicians and health-promotion specialists who are diligently working to change our thinking by promoting what they call the new weight paradigm.

- Being "thin" may not be your goal anymore. Being "healthy" is the new target.

- Accountability means traveling with others on your health journey.

First Place 4 Health in Real Life

Mark Gutierrez
California

One of my earliest memories is going to a clothing store to get some new pants when I was 4 or 5 years old. My mom was having a hard time finding pants that fit right and explained her dilemma to the sales lady. The sales lady looked at me and whispered in my mother's ear, "Why don't you try the Huskies?" I didn't know what that meant, but I figured it was bad because she whispered it. Later, I found out that I was a chubby kid, but it didn't bother me, not until I went to junior high school.

When I was 13, I went on my first diet and lost 30 pounds. The weight loss stuck with me into high school; but in college I began to diet again. Through the years I've been on countless diets. If I really tried, I was able to lose weight, but as soon as the diet was over, I would gain it all back and then some. This cycle continued until I finally gave up on ever losing weight.

In the fall of 1998, my church started offering a First Place 4 Health class. I didn't give it much thought because I had already given up on weight loss. Then I heard about a guy who lost 40 pounds on the program, and I began to wonder if it could work for me. I attended the orientation and afterward felt even more hopeless. It seemed as if those Nine Commitments would be impossible to attain. The leader was very nice and supportive, and recommended that I take the sign-up form home to pray about it. I did pray and told the Lord how tired I was of being fat and how I didn't want to try something if it wasn't going to last a lifetime. He reminded me of a video testimony about a lady who had lost more than 100 pounds and kept it off for five years. I felt a sense of hope and decided to join.

I experienced great success my first year, and as time passed, I began doing more and more of the commitments and had great support and encouragement from my leader and class members. Our group became like a family, and we would cheer each other on as we progressed toward our goals. By the end of that first year, I had developed an exercise routine that consisted of walking three to four miles five days a week. I had never exercised before, so this was a huge victory. I also quit smoking and lost 120 pounds.

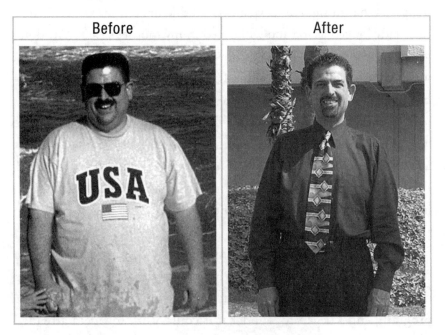

Before	After

The weight loss was great, but I quickly found that I had not developed the lifestyle that First Place talks about. You see, First Place isn't a diet; it's a lifestyle change. I still had it in my mind that I was on a diet and could go back to "normal eating" once I lost the weight. This behavior caused me to gain back almost half of my loss and I was again beginning to lose hope.

The Lord reminded me that I wasn't living a balanced life, and that's why I was experiencing weight gain. I recommitted to the program and began to lose again. During one of the Bible studies, we talked about playing old tapes in our mind. As we discussed it, I didn't think it applied to me. Then the following week I caught myself doing exactly that. I was walking by some dark windows and could see my reflection in the glass. As I saw myself, I was disgusted at my shape and began telling myself, "You're fat and ugly." I repeated that phrase in my mind several times before I realized what I was doing. I then decided to play a new tape in my mind; I told myself, "You're fit and trim."

When I considered the four-sided person—spiritual, emotional, mental and physical—I believe that I was too quick to overlook the mental side. As I trained for my first marathon, I did a lot of reading about running and training. I began to notice a theme that completing a marathon isn't just physical, but it is also mental. As a matter of fact, many believe that it's more mental than physical. You could be physically ready to run those 26.2 miles on race day, but if you don't believe that you can, you will never cross the finish line. As part of any marathon training program, there will be one long run of 20 or more miles. I've been told that it's not really necessary to run that distance in training, but you do it just so that you can convince yourself that you can run 20 miles.

I've come to realize that I'll never be successful in maintaining my weight loss if I don't begin to see myself as being that slim, healthy fellow at my goal weight. Oh, I may reach my goal weight, but if I'm not convinced that the person in the mirror is who I really am, I'll sabotage myself so that I return to that chubby fellow I believe that I am. Romans 12:2 tells us, "But let God transform you into a new person by changing the way you think" (*NLT*). Proverbs 27:3 says, "For as he thinks within himself, so he is" (*NASB*). I believe there are great truths in these Scriptures. The mind is a powerful tool; we can use it to build ourselves up, or we can use it to tear ourselves down.

I also believe that God has wonderful plans for my life, and I've allowed myself to dream about those plans. I have some dreams that are over 10 years away and would probably sound wacky to some people, but I'm convinced that it's something God wants me to do. I'm focused on those dreams and am living today so that I can be ready when it's time to fulfill those dreams.

I prayed years ago that God would use my life, my story, to share hope and encouragement to thousands; and over the years I've been given opportunities to share my story with many, many people. God has also used me to encourage a close friend. My friend Kerry has seen me go through my entire transformation. He watched as I lost those 120 pounds and quit smoking, and as I became an athlete and trained for and ran my first marathon. He joined my First Place class last year and was able to lose 14 pounds that had been plaguing him for the last decade or so. He's also gotten back into the habit of going to the gym and incorporating walks during his workday. Recently, he shared with me that my spiritual disciplines (he's aware of these because he's my accountability partner) convicted him of his need to get back on track with his quiet times.

I've come to realize that the First Place 4 Health lifestyle has to be chosen every day. It's the stuff we do day in and day out that matters over the long haul. If we veer off track for a meal, or a day, we'll be okay as long as we get right back to our healthy habits. Galatians 6:9 tells us, "So let's not get tired of doing what is good. At just the right time we will reap a harvest of blessing if we don't give up" (*NLT*). Success really is a process. If we just hang in there and keep doing what is right, we will reap the harvest.

Tim and Lynne Fast
Houston, Texas

It began on a Saturday in April 2005. I was in the kitchen and noticed the church newspaper was open to the First Place section. My wife had been trying to get me to lose weight for some time, so I jokingly said that if she wanted to join First Place, I would join with her. The next day we were at a First Place orientation meeting and signing up to start the next session. I weighed 285 pounds but was in good health, so I didn't see the need to lose weight. I figured that I could go and support my wife and maybe drop a few pounds myself.

What happened over the next 12 months was nothing short of incredible. In one year I lost 70 pounds and felt great. I no longer got winded going up stairs; my blood pressure fell to a normal range; my cholesterol dropped 50 points and my resting heart rate dropped 12 beats per minute. I hadn't been in that kind of shape for the previous 25 years!

The impact of how much weight I had lost really hit me one day while I was carrying a bag of cement on my shoulder. I was thinking how heavy it was and that it sure wasn't easy to walk with the extra weight. Then it hit me that the cement only weighed a few pounds more than the amount of weight I had lost over the previous 12 months. What an eye opener!

Losing weight makes joining First Place a positive experience for anybody, but the real benefits of joining First Place have emerged in other areas of my life.

My wife and I walk almost every evening now and have a chance to really talk to each other. It has given us the opportunity to become reacquainted after raising two sons. I have been reminded what a wonderful woman she is. We have made some very good friends in our First Place class and look forward to seeing them each week. We have memorized Scripture that will stay with us the rest of our lives, and the weekly Bible studies are great.

I thank God for the First Place program and give Him all of the credit for the changes made in my life. It's true that we can do all things through Christ who strengthens us.

Now another year has passed, and I can say again with confidence that the benefits we have received from the First Place program over the past two years have been much greater than just weight loss.

We have both grown spiritually as a result of the Bible Study and Scripture memory commitments. These commitments have led us to a deeper understanding of God's Word and His desire for us to have a more personal relationship with Him, both individually and as a couple. Lynne and I continue to feel a greater freedom to discuss our

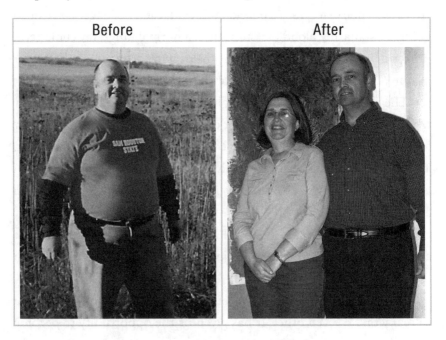

spiritual lives with each other and also to express our feelings about where we see God leading us as a couple.

The exercise commitment is where we have made the biggest change in our lives. We used to come home from work, eat supper and sit down to watch TV in the evenings. Now we come home and take a walk before we do anything else. God continues to use the time we spend walking with each other to strengthen our marriage and our commitment to Him through our marriage.

Lynne has lost and kept off 25 pounds, and I have lost 80 pounds; but the real benefit of First Place has been the growth in our spiritual lives and in our marriage.

Vicki Heath
Charleston, South Carolina

I never really struggled with my weight until after my fourth child. But I have always struggled with my self-image. After the birth of my fourth child, several things hit me at once, including some depression the realization that I was turning 40. Looking back, those two could have been related!

I heard about First Place through my mother-in-law and thought I would secretly check it out. I figured that if no one knew I was doing it, I would not have to face the failure if it didn't work out.

But it did work! I lost 25 pounds in about three sessions. As I worked through the Bible studies, God reminded me of who I am in Christ. The Lord placed in my heart a passion for leading women into a lifestyle of wellness. I launched a successful First Place ministry at my church and later became a certified fitness instructor with Body and Soul Fitness Ministries.

There are days when I still struggle with self-image and the weight issues, but most days He has the victory, and I feel very comfortable and healthy in the skin I'm in.

Megan Heath
Charleston, South Carolina

When I was about 13, my mom started in First Place. We had great meals, because she always figured out ways to cook anything in a healthy way and make it still taste good. This started my good eating habits. Mom said she wanted me to eat right in my youth instead of having to change my eating habits when I was 40.

When my mom started teaching First Place at our home church, she also wanted to try it with a high school class. Well, of course, she needed me to be in it, so I said yes. The class was a breeze. I ate what I was supposed to and I did the Bible study. But I didn't know what God was doing, because I didn't have a weight issue. But God knew that one day, food would try to spoil my self-image.

I wasn't especially pretty growing up (although mom would disagree!). I hung out with all the boys and was a typical tomboy. In college I played sports, so I was able to eat whatever I wanted, because I was very active. When I left college, I realized that I had to work at keeping a healthy body. I started running and going to aerobic classes taught by my mom. Even while doing these positive things, negative ideas began to creep into my head. I started to compare myself to people around me, even to people I didn't know, just like the teenage girls I said I would never be like.

When I got a little bit older and began to look more like a beautiful woman, my head got a little big, but God fixed that real quick! I still wanted to eat what I wanted and not worry about it. But now my plan wasn't working. So Mom and I made a pact that if something

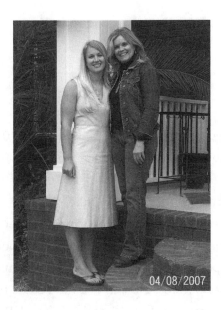

04/08/2007

wasn't "worthy," then we wouldn't eat it. I began to look at food as fuel for my tank.

I have started going back to a local First Place class. This has really helped me get back to my former good eating habits. God has showed me a lot through First Place. My body is His home, and I want it to be the best it can be while He's hanging out there. God can't use me to my fullest if I'm unhealthy and out of shape

First Place has given me a drive to take care of myself for several reasons. See if any of these hit home for you: I want to be a vessel for the King of kings; I want to be a mom who can play with her kids; I want to be a hot wife; I want to be a coach for the neighborhood team; I want to be a chaperone on a youth trip; I want to be a daughter who can care for her parents one day; I want to be a Christian others want to be like; I want to be an aunt who spoils her nieces and nephews.

These are my reasons to live a healthy life. How do you want God to use you for your expected life span?

The Fisher Family
Rockwall, Texas

Tamara's Story

Would you think you could lose 12 dress sizes and 140 pounds in a little over a year? If you answered no, then you probably feel the same way I did when I started First Place in January 2004. At that time, I was wearing a size 28 and weighed 290 pounds.

I had been overweight my whole life, starting at about the age of 10 and gradually increasing to my highest weight of 320 pounds when I got married. I was skeptical of First Place from the beginning but felt that I was running out of options. The way I saw it, I could try First Place, or undergo surgery, or get even fatter. I decided to give First Place a shot. I didn't have high expectations. I just didn't want to gain any more weight.

My whole life I had felt like a skinny person trapped in this fat body. I knew this "fat suit" I was lugging around did not fit and was not what God wanted for me. I wasn't sure if First Place was going to be the answer, but I wanted to try it and do exactly what was required. I followed all nine commitments and I was surprised every week when I lost weight. I really thought I would be the exception. I even dared the program on. I thought, *I'll do everything they say, and when it doesn't work, I'll say, "See I just can't lose weight!"* But I did.

As my heart and mind grew stronger in faith, the eating part didn't seem so tough. I kept it simple and only ate foods I knew I could count as healthy. Now I eat a wide variety of healthy foods as I've grown more confident in my choices. With an accountability partner like God, there simply was no cheating. I didn't make special allowances for birthday parties, vacations or holidays, and I didn't think I deserved a break because I did well the previous week. I just followed the program week after week.

God gave me strength when I had none and assured me it would work if I just stuck with First Place. I'm not quite at my final goal; I have about 10 pounds to go, but I know if it is His will, I will get there. My experiences represent the kind of power God can have on your life. The weight loss is just an outward expression of God's position in my life—He is first.

Weight no longer defines me. In the past, I felt that even if I was a good mother, friend or sister, I was still the fat mother, fat friend or fat sister. Now I'm just Tamara. Now I'm just me.

I am free now to live my life the way He designed it to be. I am able to reach out to people and share with them my successes through First Place. There are many examples of when my testimony of Christ's power has touched others' lives. Best of all, God is no longer a long-distance phone call or a long-lost relative I see once a year. He is my friend, and I get excited to talk to Him every day.

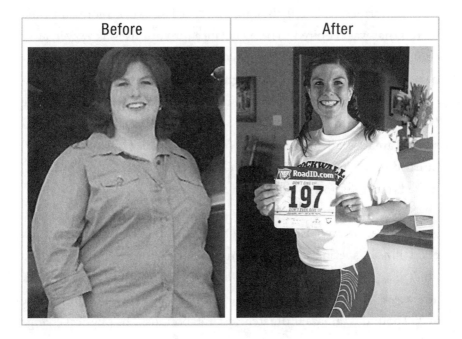

I lost 12 dress sizes and 140 pounds in a little over a year. If you were to ask me, "How did you do it?" I would simply reply, "I didn't; God did!"

I recently participated in the Rockwall Sprint Triathlon, which is a sanctioned triathlon by USA Triathlon (USAT). With a time of 1:20:38, I completed the 300-yard swim, 14-mile bike, and 3-mile run. I came in first place in Athena, second place in my age group and tenth overall female out of 120 women.

Kevin's Story

Like many other people, I was in great shape when I got married. My bride, Tamara, had struggled with her weight from an early age, but I just *knew* I could change her, and I tried. Unfortunately, it wasn't long before life changes caught up with me. I steadily gained weight up to my highest of 290 pounds, joining Tamara at her highest of 320 pounds.

As a former athlete, I thought the "eat less, work more" formula was all that was required to bring balance into our lives. However, after countless attempts with popular weight-loss diets and a few of our own, we mutually gave up on weight loss. That was until Tamara discovered First Place and committed to attending an orientation at Lake Pointe Church in Rockwall, Texas. When the day of the meeting arrived, Tamara had many excuses (including me) not to attend, and nearly didn't. Ultimately, Tamara did attend the orientation and committed to the session, which I passively supported.

Since Tamara and I never had a problem starting a weight-loss program, I knew it was just a matter of time before a birthday party, sick child, illness, special occasion or any one of a hundred situations you don't plan for would derail First Place. Decision after decision, week after week, Tamara began to change before my eyes. Starting First Place at 290 pounds, Tamara ultimately lost 140 pounds. The physical change wasn't the only thing that caught my attention, as Tamara demonstrated a spiritual and emotional maturity that astounded me.

While God worked in Tamara's life, I struggled with my faith. I grew up in church and had experiences that I related to God, but as I grew older, I did not develop my relationship with Him. I would often think, *If only there was some proof, some concrete example of God, a small personal miracle.* One day, like many in our small community, I was trying to figure out how Tamara lost the weight. It was the same formula that hadn't worked many times before, and it suddenly hit me, *You wanted a miracle.* God was the missing ingredient in the formula and He was now before me through the living testimony created in Tamara. My heart was softened, and I longed to turn my superficial understanding of God into a daily relationship. I joined First Place at the next available session.

I weighed approximately 285 pounds at that time and have since lost more than 110 pounds. I followed the nine commitments and the example set by Tamara, but the weight loss became a side effect of balance

Before	After

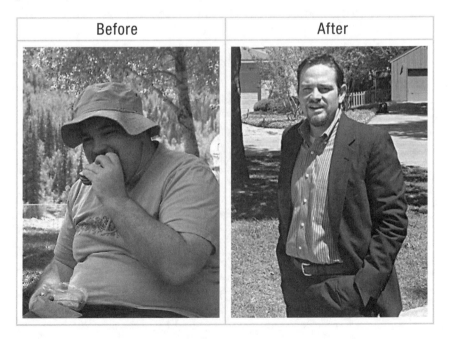

and a fruitful relationship with God. I am able to do all the activities I used to be able to do, including my favorite sports and some new activities, like run with the kids at the playground and compete in Triathlons with Tamara. Most important, I am able to do what God meant for me to do by leading my family in a balanced and spiritual manner.

I recently participated in the annual Rockwall Sprint Triathlon. I completed and posted a time of 1:17:09, which was 14 minutes faster than last year and nearly 40 minutes from when I weighed 290 pounds.

As a Couple

Tamara and I have been immensely blessed in losing 250 pounds together by following the balanced, Christ-centered program of First Place. The blessings have continued far beyond weight loss. All areas of our life have been impacted, from the physical to the spiritual. In addition, our marriage, family and friends have been inspired and changed.

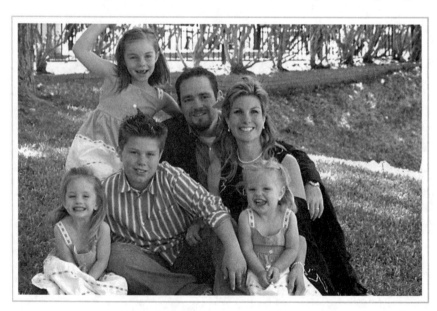

While our relationship has always been a blessing, it is stronger than ever before. As we moved closer to Christ as individuals, we found that our marriage benefited as well. Our desires had aligned and our motivations changed in a profound way as we each sought to put Christ first in our lives. Gaining health enables us to share new experiences together as we train and race in triathlons, adventure races, and running events. Crossing the finish line is an amazing experience, but crossing the finish line with your spouse is an even greater experience. And as Mom and Dad, we are better equipped to teach our four children many valuable lessons.

Today our family leads an active, healthy, spiritually alive lifestyle. We talk about the foods we eat, the decisions we make and the long-term impact they can have on our body. We encourage quiet time, biblical learning and fellowship with friends and family. We enjoy television and video games, but we also enjoy soccer and cycling. In addition to an active lifestyle, our two oldest children recently joined us in a 20-mile urban-adventure race. Such an accomplishment was a confidence boost for the entire family and we have plans to compete in additional races in the future. God's role in our life is evident to those around us and we are eager to share His story.

Numerous friends have been inspired to join First Place and now have great testimonies themselves. In addition, Tamara's mother and sisters have also joined with great results. Alexi, my sister-in-law, started First Place wearing a size 16 and now wears a size 6. Marvin, my brother, lost approximately 60 pounds through the First Place lifestyle.

Our family has been forever changed as we strive to place Christ first in our life.

Chapter 12

Putting It All Together

Today you are embarking on a journey.

You are ready to take the next steps toward living a balanced life. That life is a good life, the life God wants you to live. He designed you to live that way. When your life is balanced, you will be able to fully enjoy and embrace every opportunity God brings your way.

It's always easy whenever you read a book to finish the last page, shut the book and never take action on what you've just read.

But think back to your motivations for losing weight that you wrote about in the beginning chapters of this book. Do you want to be healthy? Do you want to be well? Do you want to be able to pick up your children, or not be winded when you play with your grand-children? Perhaps one of your parents died too young from a prevent-able disease, and you don't want to make that mistake. Perhaps a friend or loved one is living a long but unhappy life because of poor choices he or she has made along the way—and you want to follow a different path.

Keeping your goal in mind is so crucial to your success. A goal is a dream with a timeline. Develop your goal. Know your goal. Keep it in mind. Remind yourself again and again why living an imbalanced life is not an option for you anymore.

Sometimes our goal seems relatively small, even humorous. All that my friend Joe Ann Winkler wanted to do initially was to be able to "walk faster than an 80-year-old man."

Joe Ann had developed multiple sclerosis as a 16-year-old in 1950. Because of the disease, she was only able to walk short distances. Over the years she was fitted for leg braces and often used a wheelchair. At most, she could only walk a few steps. Because of her medical condition and the resulting sedentary lifestyle, she became overweight.

In her late 50s, Joe Ann joined First Place. Steroid use wreaked havoc on her metabolism, but Joanne was determined to make healthy choices. Pounds came and went. Sometimes they came back again because of her medications.

Joe Ann bought a bracelet with the words "believe," "trust" and "obey" inscribed on it. She wanted to believe that she could lose weight, trust God to help her, and obey His direction for her life. Joe Ann found inspiration in Philippians 4:13: "I can do everything through him who gives me strength."

Joe Ann determined to walk more than a few steps. She believed that God could give her the ability to do so. Joe Ann knew she had to act on her faith, so she started walking a few steps every day. Each day she walked just a bit more. When it rained, she walked at the mall. She walked at a snail's pace. Everybody passed her. Her goal became to pass just one person. Finally she did—she passed an 80-year-old man with a cane. It wasn't much, she said, but at least it was something.

Joe Ann kept up with her walking. She set more goals—of walking one mile, then two. She began to pray as she walked. Even in the mall, she would silently pray for people she saw in the mall. People began to remark that her walking was becoming stronger.

Today Joe Ann regularly walks three miles every morning. She has lost 77 pounds, and her commitment to the Lord is stronger than ever.

She started small and developed her goal. She knew her goal and kept it in mind. She reminded herself again and again why living an imbalanced life was not an option for her anymore. And she succeeded.

And you can, too!

A Dream with a Timeline

I know that it can be daunting to look ahead to the end of your goal in light of where you are today. Some people get discouraged before even beginning. Don't make that mistake!

Just take it one day at a time. Just for today, ask the Lord to give you the best day possible. Just for today. Then do it again tomorrow, and the day after that. Do the next right thing. Make your next meal a healthy meal. Take a walk to the corner and back. Before you go to bed tonight, do one healthy thing for yourself, even if it's just praying for five minutes. Begin to put in place what you're going to do.

Let's look back over some of the things we've discussed in this book, and see if we can put it all together.

We talked about how we're a nation fixated on weight loss, but 95 percent of people who lose weight gain it back. Why? We want instant solutions, not real-life change. First, we looked at some of the history of First Place and why it is a program with a long track record of success that can be trusted.

We also discussed how you won't find the solution to your health needs overnight but you will learn to live healthily for the rest of your life. At First Place 4 Health, our challenge to you is to give us a year. Give us one year, and we'll show you a lasting plan to lose weight and gain health and wholeness.

We mentioned how God didn't promise us that life would be rosy and without difficulty. Instead, the Lord promised to carry us through any situation and any trial. Weight loss will happen in your life—you can do it, but it won't happen without some effort. The Lord knows the obstacles and excuses that come up. But quitting isn't the answer. To begin your education to a new lifestyle, you need to show up. That means getting on the bus.

First place is not a diet program, but a lifestyle change. The goal is living a balanced life, spiritually, mentally, emotionally and physically.

There are two biblical foundational components to grasp as you begin your journey: (1) You have the power to decide to live a healthier life; and (2) true, lasting change happens through the power of the Holy Spirit.

A true lifestyle change is something that happens best with the help of a trusted group of friends. It's very hard to change by yourself. The First Place program provides the small group to help you along. But of all the invitations in the program, the first is the strongest: You've got to show up. In a First Place 4 Health group, you'll learn the ins and outs of the program. You'll also find the tools, support and encouragement to help you along the way.

It sounds almost ironic that when you show up each week at your group meeting, you're asked to show up and encourage somebody. When you enter with this mindset, it actually benefits you. Other people need your encouragement as much as you need theirs. When you show up with the purpose of encouraging others, it can make all the difference.

When people think of weight loss, they automatically think of physical changes. But lasting change starts when you begin to ingest truth into your life. This happens when you meet with God daily through His Word.

Reading God's Word each day is like a light snack for your spirit. Studying God's Word is like a real meal. Each week, First Place 4 Health participants are invited to study the Bible in practical ways with the help of their small group.

Prayer is so important to your spiritual balance. It's where you talk to God and God also talks to you. Prayer is a regular part of your balanced life.

What you think affects how you act. When you truly get the Word of God in your mind, you receive the very thoughts of God. Memorizing Scripture isn't easy for everybody, but we explored why it's so necessary, and we gave some helpful hints to make this a part of your journey toward a balanced life.

We talked about how First Place is not a diet. We won't put you on a restrictive plan of celery and tofu. At First Place 4 Health, we believe in enjoying all the nutritional foods that the Lord has given us. This means eating quality foods in the right quantity. We'll show you what this means in depth at the weekly meetings.

God designed your body to move, and you can't live a balanced life by sitting around all day. Exercise includes daily lifestyle activity as well as cardiovascular, strength and flexibility training. You may have never exercised a day in your life, but we want to help you create a plan that fits your needs. You'll begin to see the benefits almost immediately.

And finally, we talked about how First Place 4 Health encourages accountability. Success is seldom achieved alone. We help you build success into every component of living a balanced life. And we'll give you practical tools at our weekly meetings that will help you do that.

Your Next Step

A balanced life is a gift to yourself. It's your choice to live a balanced life. No one can make that choice for you. Start now. Imagine your future both ways—if you choose to be healthy or choose not to be. With God's help, you have the power to decide the outcome.

As with any journey, there will be setbacks. But a journey means that you are going forward. You're making progress in the right direction. Determine that you're not going to quit. Resolve to stay strong until the end of the journey.

You may think this journey is all about losing weight, but God knows and cares about everything that happens in your life. He wants you to be a whole person—spiritually, mentally, emotionally and physically. First Place 4 Health is not just a weight-loss program; it's about the total person. It's about learning to give Christ first place in every area so that He can make the necessary changes in your life.

What's the immediate invitation in front of you today? Just give us a year.

Your year starts here.

Write down today's date: _____

Give us one year, and allow God to work the way He wants to work in your life. It's not just about losing weight. It's about a lifestyle change. True, First Place 4 Health teaches you how to deal with your weight—but that's a side benefit. At its core, First Place 4 Health teaches you how to give Christ first place so that you learn how to truly live.

Your specific choice today is simple: It's whether or not to say yes. Are you willing to start on this path to living a balanced life? Even—are you willing to let God show you what it means to be willing?

In front of you today is the beginning of a brand-new life. When you journey down this road, you're going to find out who God really is—and how wonderful He is. His desire is to make you into the person He wants you to be from the day you were born. And that person is wonderful. God always has something so much better for us! It's never that He wants to punish us by not letting us have cookies. It's that He wants us to have the abundant life He promises.

Are you willing to join me on this exciting journey of change? My promise to you is that if you won't quit, you will succeed. Success is found in the process, not in a program. And permanent lifestyle changes don't happen quickly. But they will happen.

Give us one year.

You will begin to lose the weight you want. You'll get the balance in your life you need. And you'll find health, healing and wholeness along the way.

Beyond the Basics

First Place website: www.firstplace.org

A variety of resources can be found at the First Place 4 Health website. Find information about upcoming events, networking opportunities, bulletin boards, recipes, stories, and more. First Place 4 Health leaders can find all the resources they need to start, promote and lead a group. Members share their success stories to inspire and encourage you. Find the history of the program and full descriptions of various program aspects. Find First Place books, Bible studies and other supplementary products.

First Place 4 Health Conferences

Once you've learned the basic program of First Place 4 Health, you have learned the foundational elements. But First Place 4 Health is a program much broader than the initial groups.

First Place 4 Health conferences are held throughout the year in different locations, such as Nashville, New Orleans, Cincinnati or Dallas. There are no prerequisites to attending a First Place 4 Health conference. Some of the participants are leaders in First Place who want to receive additional training, while others simply want to learn more about the program. Leaders and their class members often attend these events to enrich their lives spiritually, emotionally, mentally and physically.

Many people who attend our conferences have never been in First Place 4 Health but want to learn about the program. Conference participants attend a wide selection of seminars that address spiritual and emotional growth, as well as seminars that teach members how to take care of their bodies. They will also enjoy hearing a number of dynamic speakers.

The atmosphere at these conferences is electric, and the fellowship with other Christians is a boost to your spiritual life. An added plus is the opportunity to eat First Place 4 Health meals and discover first-hand how wonderful these recipes can be. For specific dates and times, check the First Place 4 Health website: www.firstplace4health.org.

First Place 4 Health Spa Weeks

In addition to the First Place 4 Health conferences, several times a year we offer a Spa Week program at Round Top, Texas. The times and speakers vary. The week-long conference includes inspirational messages, exercise time, praise and worship, and devotionals. These in-depth meetings give participants a chance to interact with various leaders of First Place 4 Health and get their questions and concerns answered individually. More than anything else, these Spa Weeks are spiritual experiences that boost the life of each participant.

Spa Week includes:

• *Daily Bible Study and Devotionals.* Each day, we gather together for a morning devotional and prayer time led by First Place 4 Health leaders. During this time, we study the Bible using the latest First Place 4 Health Bible study. Later in the day, we meet in small groups to get to know each other better and pray for our challenges and concerns.

• *Exercise for Every Fitness Level.* Activities include aerobics, strength and endurance training, stretching, power walking, biking, Pilates, and interval training for those who think they "can't exercise." Each activity is designed to meet the fitness level of each individual, and participation is optional.

- *Delicious First Place 4 Health Meals.* Enjoy healthy meals made from the freshest ingredients. You will be amazed at the delicious, satisfying meals you can have using First Place 4 Health recipes. All the recipes will be provided for you to take home and try yourself. Your meal may include Johnny's Cajun Meatloaf, Chicken Supreme with mushroom gravy and wild rice, Pumpkin Soufflé, Apple Dumplings, and more. Breakfast is served continental style with healthy options, such as yogurt, fruit, cereal and toast.

- *Rest and Relaxation.* Porch Time is a favorite activity at Round Top. Talking and relaxing with friends on the porch is on the schedule every afternoon. Benches are dispersed around the grounds for you to sit and read, have your quiet time or just relax. The scent of clean, country air and the sounds of wildlife and nature surround you in this peaceful, serene setting.

- *Complete Fitness Testing.* This includes body composition, cholesterol, glucose, blood pressure, aerobic capacity, flexibility, and more. Trinity Medical Center will have nursing staff at the retreat center who will administer the testing. You will be given a health report with complete directions for understanding your results and tips for improving your health. If you have attended Spa Week before, you will also receive a progress report comparing your previous results.

- *Praise and Worship Times.*

- *Inspirational Speakers.*

- *Pamper Yourself.* During the week, a certified relaxation massage therapist is available. Pamper yourself with a relaxing massage after your workout or before you go to bed. A certified nail technician will also be available for manicures, pedicures and nail treatments.

First Place 4 Health One-Day Workshops

If you want additional help learning the First Place 4 Health program or want to know how to begin and lead a First Place 4 Health group or program in your church or community, call our office to find out about a workshop in your area.

One-day workshops are now offered all around the country. The purpose of the workshop is a passion to see the ministry grow. Each one is hosted by a church with an active First Place 4 Health program. The workshops teach such topics as the history of the program, the four-sided goals, the mechanics of starting a program, what it takes to be a leader, meeting procedures, and the food plan.

A First Place 4 Health workshop may be a good way to learn more about First Place 4 Health and to give you the tools to begin a program where you live. Workshops are usually held on a Saturday from 9:00 A.M. to 2:00 P.M.

Advanced Training for Leaders

Once a year we hold a two-day leadership summit welcoming First Place 4 Health leaders from around the nation. All the workshops, brainstorming sessions, and special teaching times will center on instruction, inspiration and motivation. The Leadership Summit is held at Houston's First Baptist Church the last Friday and Saturday in July.

Spend an incredible two days of celebrating, networking, brainstorming, idea sharing, praying, training and worship. All First Place 4 Health networking leaders, workshop leaders, active, former and potential leaders are invited to attend. Sample workshops include:

- Leadership Accountability
- Building Your Ministry
- Exercise Accountability
- Beginning Leader Training
- Leading the Live It Plan
- Creative Leadership
- Community Connections
- Nutrition and Fitness
- Plus more!

Monthly E-Newsletter Resource

First Place 4 Health also has a monthly e-newsletter that provides inspiration, motivational articles, fitness information, recipes, articles about nutrition and fitness, as well as conference, Fitness Week and workshop information. Each month's issue features an inspiring testimony with before and after photos. The newsletter is available free online. To subscribe, log on to www.firstplace.org.

Area Leaders' Meetings

Area Leaders' Meetings are scheduled by First Place 4 Health networking leaders who are eager to help, support and encourage you in your First Place 4 Health ministry. Some of the goals of these meetings are:

- Sharing common struggles and finding solutions
- Passing on successful strategies
- Sharing new ideas

If you would be interested in attending an Area Leaders' Meeting, please contact the networking leader nearest you. First Place Networking Leaders may be found at www.firstplace4health.org.

Choosing Christ

The most important choice you will ever make is the decision to put Christ first in your life. If you have not already made that commitment, prayerfully read the following verses that explain what it means to become a Christian, and how to do so.

Becoming a Christian

God is a holy God, and He shows us a perfect standard of righteousness. When we read passages of Scripture such as the Ten Commandments (see Exodus 20:1-18), we know that we can never keep all of the commandments perfectly. We begin to see ourselves as lawbreakers—as sinners.

> I would not have known what sin was except through the law. For I would not have known what coveting really was if the law had not said, "Do not covet" (Romans 7:7).

Have you ever told a lie? Have you ever cheated or lusted or dishonored your parents or cursed someone using God's name? God looks upon the attitudes of our heart as well as our actions. God is a holy God and cannot have anything to do with our sin. All of mankind in sinful and separated from God.

> All have sinned and fall short of the glory of God (Romans 3:23).

The wages of our sin is death—or separation from God. God says that hell is a reality. We will all die one day, and God cannot have anything to do with sin.

The wages of sin is death, but the gift of God is eternal life in Christ Jesus our Lord (Romans 6:23).

Many people try to get close to God by doing good things or going to church. But simply trying to be a good person is not the answer. Jesus said He is the only way to God.

I am the way and the truth and the life. No one comes to the Father except through me (John 14:6).

The Bible says the only way to God is through His Son, Jesus Christ, who died on the cross for you and me. That's a gift available to us by grace—it's not anything we deserve or earn. Salvation is freely given to us when we ask Jesus for it.

For it is by grace you have been saved, through faith—and this not from yourselves, it is the gift of God—not by works, so that no one can boast (Ephesians 2:8-9).

God gives you salvation as a free gift. A gift must be accepted. Our invitation is to accept Christ.

Everyone who calls on the name of the Lord will be saved (Romans 10:13).

God loves you and offers you everlasting life. Salvation is available to everyone who believes. This is the wonderful news of the gospel.

For God so loved the world that he gave His one and only son, that whoever believes in him shall not perish but have everlasting life (John 3:16).

How can you be sure you're saved? Scripture asks us one short question: Do you have Christ? There is much confidence in knowing that when you have Christ, you are indeed saved.

> God has given us eternal life, and this life is in his Son. He who has the Son has life; he who does not have the Son of God does not have life. I write these things to you who believe in the name of the Son of God so that you may know that you have eternal life (1 John 5:11-13).

When we become Christians, Jesus will give us the "fruit of the Spirit" as we yield to God and the Holy Spirit begins to work in our lives. Jesus gives us this peace and joy, etc., as a result of our salvation.

> The fruit of the Spirit is love, joy, peace, patience, kindness, goodness, faithfulness, gentleness and self-control (Galatians 5:22-23).

Once we are saved, God asks us to grow and mature in our faith. We are saved for a reason—to serve and glorify God.

> For we are God's workmanship, created in Christ Jesus to do good works, which God prepared in advance for us to do (Ephesians 2:10).

Spiritually, where do you stand today? Do you know for certain that if you died tonight you would be with Christ in heaven? If not, why not turn to Christ right now. I invite you to pray this prayer. It doesn't matter the words you use. What matters is the attitude of your heart.

Jesus, I know that You are a holy and righteous God. I know that I am a sinner and separated from You. Thank You for loving me and dying on the cross for me. Please forgive me of my sins and help me to give my life totally to You. Please come into my life and be my Lord and Savior. Amen.

Steps for Spiritual Growth

When you become a Christian, God invites you to grow in your faith. Some actions that will help in this area include:

- *Reading the Bible* keeps you grounded in God's Word for your daily choices about how you will live.

- *Praying* gives you the opportunity to communicate with God and for Him to communicate with you.

- *Attending church* provides fellowship with other believers, a place to learn more about God, and opportunities for service to other believers and to the world.

- *Worshiping* gives you the opportunity to tell God that there is nothing and no one more important than Him. Worship can happen any time. You can worship God when you're alone or when you're with others, praising God together.

- *Serving* is an expression of your gratitude to God and your trust in Him. It is a result of your changed heart and priorities.

- *Witnessing.* When you put your trust in Christ as your Savior and Lord, you will want to tell others about the good news of Christ and what He has done for all who will come to Him.

About the Author and Collaborative Author

Carole Lewis is the national director of First Place 4 Health, the Christ-centered health and weight-loss program. A warm, transparent and humorous communicator, Carole is a popular speaker at workshops, seminars and conferences around the country. Carole has been on staff at Houston's First Baptist Church since 1984, and has written 10 books. She and her husband, Johnny, have three adult children (one deceased), eight grandchildren, and one great-grandchild. They live in the Galveston Bay area of Texas, near Houston, where their favorite pastime is sitting on the pier and watching the sunset.

Marcus Brotherton is a professional writer, and the author or coauthor of 17 books. He holds a master's degree from Talbot Seminary at Biola University and a bachelor's degree from Multnomah Bible College. He lives with his wife and daughter in Washington State.

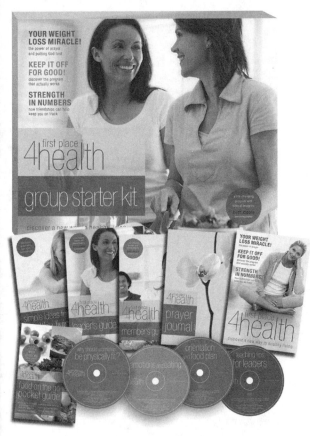
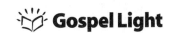

4 first place health

discover a new way to healthy living

CHANGE YOUR LIFE FOREVER BY PUTTING CHRIST FIRST!

Start Today with These First Place 4 Health Bible Studies

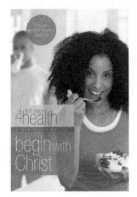

Begin with Christ
The first in a new series of Bible studies for the First Place 4 Health program, *Begin with Christ* will help members focus on surrendering to God.

ISBN 10-digit: 08307.45181
ISBN 13-digit: 978.08307.45180

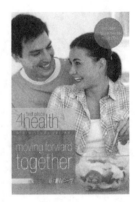

Moving Forward Together
Give participants new inspiration to focus on the journey of following Christ and living according to His guidelines.

ISBN 10-digit: 08307.45203
ISBN 13-digit: 978.08307.45203

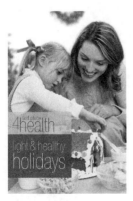

Light & Healthy Holidays
Provides staying power during the tempting holiday season and encouragement to reflect on the true reason for the holidays.

ISBN 10-digit: 08307.46730
ISBN 13-digit: 978.08307.46736

Available at bookstores everywhere or by calling 1-800-4-GOSPEL.
Join the First Place 4 Health community and order products at
www.firstplace4health.com

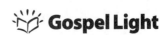 **Gospel Light**

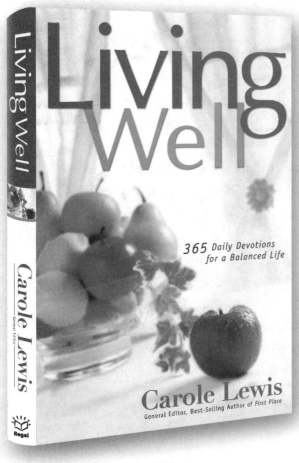
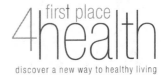
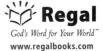

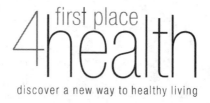

discover a new way to healthy living

For more information about
First Place 4 Health,
please contact:

First Place 4 Health
7401 Katy Freeway
Houston, TX 77024
1-800-72-PLACE (727-5223)
email: info@firstplace4health.org
website: www.firstplace4health.org